The Optic Nerve Evaluation in Glaucoma

AN INTERACTIVE WORKBOOK

The Optic Nerve Evaluation in Glaucoma

AN INTERACTIVE WORKBOOK

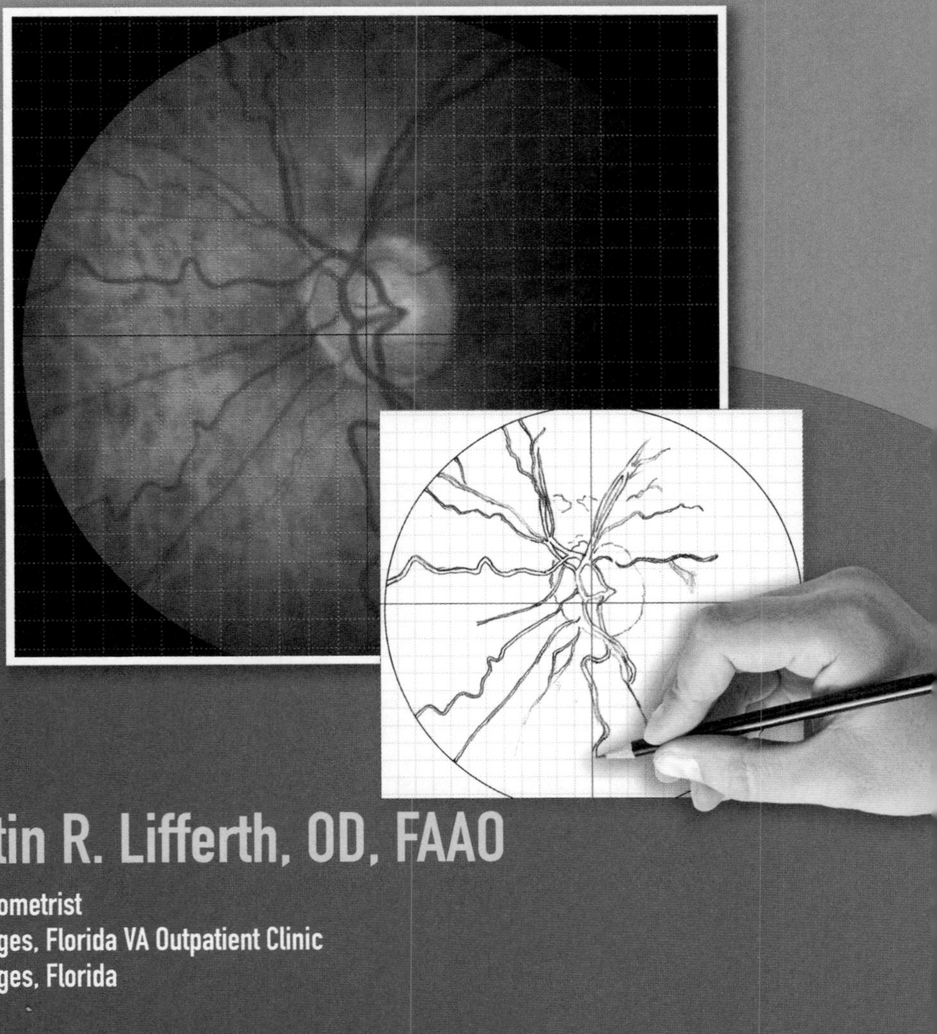

Austin R. Lifferth, OD, FAAO

Staff Optometrist
The Villages, Florida VA Outpatient Clinic
The Villages, Florida

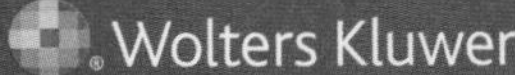

Philadelphia • Baltimore • New York • London
Buenos Aires • Hong Kong • Sydney • Tokyo

Acquisitions Editor: Chris Teja
Senior Development Editor: Kristina Oberle
Editorial Coordinator: LaRae Price
Marketing Manager: Rachel Mante Leung
Production Project Manager: David Orzechowski
Design Coordinator: Stephen Druding
Manufacturing Coordinator: Beth Welsh
Prepress Vendor: S4Carlisle Publishing Services

9 8 7 6 5 4 3 2 1

Printed in China

Library of Congress Cataloging-in-Publication Data

Names: Lifferth, Austin R., author.
Title: The optic nerve evaluation in glaucoma : an interactive workbook / Austin R. Lifferth, OD, FAAO, Staff Optometrist, The Villages, Florida VA Outpatient Clinic.
Description: Philadelphia: Wolters Kluwer, [2017] | Includes bibliographical references and index.
Identifiers: LCCN 2017005550 | ISBN 9781496363138
Subjects: LCSH: Glaucoma—Diagnosis.
Classification: LCC RE871 .L55 2017 | DDC 617.7/410754—dc23 LC record available at https://lccn.loc.gov/2017005550

Acknowledgments

I gratefully acknowledge my professors at Indiana University School of Optometry who helped me *discover* my interest in glaucoma. I will be forever indebted to Matthew Cordes OD, Lee Peplinski OD, and many other outstanding mentors within the eye care profession who have helped me *develop* my interest in glaucoma. I am grateful to my patients, who continually encourage me to *deepen* my interest in glaucoma.

Contents

Preface

I recall taking a "surprise quiz" related to glaucoma early in my education while at Indiana University School of Optometry—and performing somewhat poorly.

Ironically, and in retrospect, I am grateful for that shocking self-assessment. In fact, from that singular defining moment, an unexpected catalyst was created to learn more and understand more about glaucoma. As a result of this delightful process over the years, I have learned to better appreciate the characteristic clinical signs of glaucoma and also the surprising subtleties of glaucoma.

More specific on how to evaluate the optic nerve in glaucoma, this interactive workbook is an informal attempt to share "what I wish I had known more" when I started my profession over a decade ago. Hopefully, your active learning within this workbook will be an excellent review and a timely reminder of how to systematically evaluate the optic nerve in glaucoma—a foundational (yet perishable) skill that may be progressively underutilized by eye care providers and overshadowed by advancing technology.

1. INTRODUCTION

Glaucoma, despite its multifactorial etiology, is an optic neuropathy with characteristic quantitative and qualitative optic nerve defects.[1]

Over the past few decades, numerous authors[2–9] have identified several key quantitative and qualitative optic nerve features that should be *systematically* evaluated for and considered in every patient. These characteristic morphologic features include the following:

- **a.** Optic disc size
- **b.** Optic disc shape
- **c.** Optic cup shape and depth
- **d.** Optic cup size in relation to the optic disc size
- **e.** Neuroretinal rim size, shape, and perfusion
- **f.** Central retinal vessel trunk location
- **g.** Optic disc hemorrhages
- **h.** Parapapillary chorioretinal atrophy
- **i.** Retinal arteriole diameter
- **j.** Retinal nerve fiber layer defects

Regarding these characteristic features, it is interesting to note that almost all *quantitative* variables (e.g., cup-disc diameter and area ratios) have broad overlap between normal patients and glaucoma patients.[3]

Conversely, *qualitative* variables such as visible retinal nerve fiber layer defects and disc hemorrhages have a higher specificity in separating glaucomatous eyes from nonglaucomatous eyes in the proper clinical setting.[3]

Furthermore, although some of these features may be found in isolation, others may be combined with other characteristic features—and are not necessarily sequential with respect to each other.

As eye care providers, it is critically important for each of us to *habitually identify* and *clinically interpret* these quantitative and qualitative optic nerve defects in glaucoma to make a more accurate and timely diagnosis. Regrettably, for a chronic disease that is mostly relatively asymptomatic, these early defects may be underdiagnosed, overdiagnosed. . .or just plain misdiagnosed.

The purpose of this workbook is twofold:

1. Learn to *habitually identify* the above quantitative and qualitative variables during our *routine* exams.
2. Consistently *clinically interpret* these quantitative and qualitative variables during our *glaucoma* exams.

To help achieve this purpose, this workbook has two main complementary sections.

First, within each main section, there is a brief and factual overview of each key topic with associated clinical pearls.

Second, within each correlating section, there are images that represent the associated clinical features as well as a unique opportunity to draw or sketch those features. In short, if a picture is worth a thousand words, then drawing it will be worth so much more as it adds to our awareness, attention, and accuracy of those characteristic features.

Hopefully the mental process of reviewing these characteristic features, combined with the biomechanical process of drawing these features, will have a synergistic effect of deepening our understanding and sharpening our individual diagnostic skills. . .

Enjoy!
Austin

References

1. Weinreb R, Aung T, Medeiros F. The pathophysiology and treatment of glaucoma: a review. *JAMA*. 2014;311(18):1901–1911.
2. Armaly M, Sayegh R. The cup-disc ratio. The findings of tonometry and tonography in the normal eye. *Arch Ophthalmol.* 1969;82(2):191–196.
3. Jonas J, Budde W, Panda-Jonas S. Ophthalmoscopic evaluation of the optic nerve head. *Surv Ophthalmol.* 1999;43:293–320.
4. Broadway D, Nicolela M, Drance S. Optic disk appearances in primary open-angle glaucoma. *Surv Ophthalmol.* 1999;43(suppl 1):S223–S243.
5. Spaeth GL, Henderer J, Liu C, et al. The disc damage likelihood scale: reproducibility of a new method of estimating the amount of optic nerve damage caused by glaucoma. *Trans Am Ophthalmol Soc.* 2002;100:181–185; discussion 185–186.
6. Fingeret M, Medeiros F, Susanna R Jr, et al. Five rules to evaluate the optic disc and retinal nerve fiber layer for glaucoma. *Optometry.* 2005;76:661–668.
7. Susanna R, Medeiros FA. *The Optic Nerve in Glaucoma*. 2nd ed. Rio de Janeiro, Brazil: Cultura Medica; 2006.
8. Susanna R, Vessani R. New findings in the evaluation of the optic disc in glaucoma diagnosis. *Curr Opin Ophthalmol.* 2007;18(2):122–128.
9. Jonas J, Bergua A, Schmitz-Valckenberg P, et al. Ranking of optic disc variables for detection of glaucomatous optic nerve damage. *Invest Ophthalmol Vis Sci.* 2000;41(7):1764–1773.

2. OPTIC DISC SIZE

Overview

Careful and systematic evaluation of the optic nerve for glaucoma *first* begins with accurately determining the size of the optic disc. Correcting for optic disc size provides clinical context to cup-disc ratio, rim-disc ratio, and neuroretinal rim area measurements to help us diagnose glaucoma earlier and detect progression sooner.[1]

Pearls

- **Optic disc size correlates with the optic cup size and the neuroretinal rim area.**[2]
    - The larger the optic disc size, the larger the cup and the neuroretinal rim.
        - A large cup in a large optic disc may be normal *and* a small or average cup in a small disc may suggest glaucomatous optic nerve damage.
        - The cup-disc ratio can range from 0.0 to 0.9 in the normal population with significant overlap between normal and glaucomatous eyes.[3]
        - Careful examination of the vertical cup-disc ratio *corrected for disc size* increases specificity and sensitivity.[4]
        - Number of retinal nerve fibers in normal eyes is variable and ranges from 750,000 to 1.5 million.[5]
            - Larger nerves may have more retinal nerve fibers.[6,7]
- **Significant intrapopulation and interpopulation variability.**
    - Age: disc area independent of age beyond 3 to 10 years of age.[8,9]
        - Prevalence of glaucoma increases with age.[10]
    - Gender: No statistically significant difference or consensus.[8]
    - Body length/weight: inconclusive in some studies, but others report increased disc area of 0.02 mm^2 with each 10-cm increase in body length for normal body height.[2]
    - Refractive error: within –5 to +5 D, statistically independent[9]; other studies suggested that disc area linearly increased by 1.2% +/–0.15% for each diopter toward myopia.[2]
        - Higher hyperopia (>+5): smaller disc than emmetropic eyes.[2]
        - Higher myopia (>–8): larger, elongated disc than emmetropic eyes.[11]
    - Race: "one may infer that the disc size increases with ethnically determined pigmentation"[2]—i.e., African Americans > Asians > Hispanics > Caucasians.

    - Mean disc area[1]:
      - African Americans: 2.14–3.75 mm^2
      - Asians: 2.47–3.22 mm^2
      - Hispanics: 2.46–2.67 mm^2
      - Caucasians: 1.73–2.63 mm^2

- **Morphogenetic implications[2]:**
  - Larger optic discs (as compared to smaller optic discs) have:
    - Larger neuroretinal rim area.
    - More optic nerve fibers.[6,7]
      - Smaller optic discs may have a smaller anatomic reserve capacity.
    - More lamina cribrosa pores/area.
    - Less nerve fiber crowding per mm^2 of disc area.
    - Great number of cilioretinal arteries.

- **Pathogenetic implications:**
  - Small discs: more commonly have optic disc drusen, pseudopapilledema, nonarteritic ischemic optic neuropathy.[12,13]
    - Small discs with glaucomatous cupping may still be underdiagnosed because of the relative lower cup-disc ratios.
  - Large discs: more commonly may have optic nerve pits and morning glory syndrome.[2]
    - Variable consensus on increased glaucoma susceptibility.[14,15]
      - Large discs with expected larger cupping may be overdiagnosed because of the relative higher cup-disc ratios.
  - Normal discs: more commonly have arteritic and retinal vascular occlusions, primary open-angle glaucoma (including juvenile-onset) and secondary open-angle glaucoma (pigmentary > pseudoexfoliation).[2]

- **Measurement of the optic disc size[2]:**
  - Clinical assessment:
    - Identify the optic disc limits as all of the area *inside* of the peripapillary scleral ring.
      - Peripapillary scleral ring does not belong to the optic disc.
      - Including the peripapillary scleral ring into the disc area:
        - Will increase the neuroretinal rim area.
        - Will decrease the cup-disc ratio.
        - May underestimate the *real* damage and undertreat the patient.
    - Adjust slit lamp beam length to match the vertical diameter of the optic disc, read on graticule with respective correction factor.
      - Fundus lens correction factor:
        - VolK: 60 D (0.88×), 66 D (1.0×), 78 D (1.2×), 90 D (1.33×).
        - Nikon: 60 D (1.03×), 90 D (1.63×).
      - Disc size: small (<1.5 mm), medium (1.5–2.0 mm), large (>2.0 mm).[16,17]

References

1. Hoffmann EM, Zangwill LM, Crowston JG, et al. Optic disk size and glaucoma. *Surv Ophthalmol.* 2007;52(1):32–49.
2. Jonas JB, Budde WM, Panda-Jonas S. Ophthalmoscopic evaluation of the optic nerve head. *Surv Ophthalmol.* 1999;43:293–320.
3. Jonas JB, Gusek GC, Naumann GO. Optic disc, cup and neuroretinal rim size, configuration and correlations in normal eyes. *Invest Ophthalmol Vis Sci.* 1988;29:1151–1158.
4. Jonas JB, Bergua A, Schmitz-Valckenberg P, et al. Ranking of optic disc variables for detection of glaucomatous optic nerve damage. *Invest Ophthalmol Vis Sci.* 2000;41:1764–1773.
5. Jonas JB, Schmidt AM, Müller-Bergh JA, et al. Human optic nerve fiber count and optic disc size. *Invest Ophthalmol Vis Sci.* 1992;33:2012–2018.
6. Quigley HA, Coleman AL, Dorman-Pease ME. Larger optic nerve heads have more nerve fibers in normal monkey eyes. *Arch Ophthalmol.* 1991;109:1441–1443.
7. Yucel YH, Gupta N, Kalichman MW, et al. Relationship of optic disc topography to optic nerve fiber number in glaucoma. *Arch Ophthalmol.* 1998;116:493–497.
8. Varma R, Tielsch JM, Quigley HA, et al. Race-, age-, gender-, and refractive error-related differences in the normal optic disc. *Arch Ophthalmol.* 1994;112:1068–1076.
9. Bowd C, Zangwill LM, Blumenthal EZ, et al. Imaging of the optic disc and retinal nerve fiber layer: the effects of age, optic disc area, refractive error, and gender. *J Opt Soc Am A Opt Image Sci Vis.* 2002;19:197–207.
10. Klein BE, Klein R, Sponsel WE, et al. Prevalence of glaucoma. The Beaver Dam Eye Study. *Ophthalmology.* 1992;99:1499–1504.
11. Jonas JB, Gusek GC, Naumann GO. Optic disk morphometry in high myopia. *Graefes Arch Clin Exp Ophthalmol.* 1988;226:587–590.
12. Jonas JB. Frequency of optic disc drusen and size of the optic disc. *Ophthalmology.* 1997;104:1531–1532.
13. Jonas JB, Gusek GC, Naumann GO. Anterior ischemic optic neuropathy: nonarteritic form in small and giant cell arteritis in normal sized optic discs. *Int Ophthalmol.* 1988;12:119–125.
14. Zangwill LM, Weinreb RN, Beiser JA, et al. Baseline topographic optic disc measurements are associated with the development of primary open-angle glaucoma: the Confocal Scanning Laser Ophthalmoscopy Ancillary Study to the Ocular Hypertension Treatment Study. *Arch Ophthalmol.* 2005;123:1188–1197.
15. Jonas JB, Fernández MC, Naumann GO. Correlation of the optic disc size to glaucoma susceptibility. *Ophthalmology.* 1991;98:675–680.
16. Spaeth GL, Henderer J, Liu C, et al. The disc damage likelihood scale: reproducibility of a new method of estimating the amount of optic nerve damage caused by glaucoma. *Trans Am Ophthalmol Soc.* 2002;100:181–185; discussion 185–186.
17. Henderer J, Liu C, Spaeth G, et al. Original articles: reliability of the disk damage likelihood scale. *Am J Ophthalmol.* 2003;135:44–48.

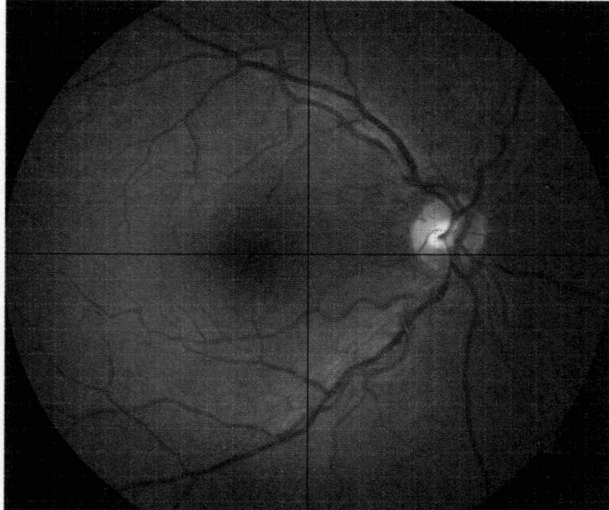

Average-small nerve with healthy and even retinal nerve fiber layer pattern distribution.

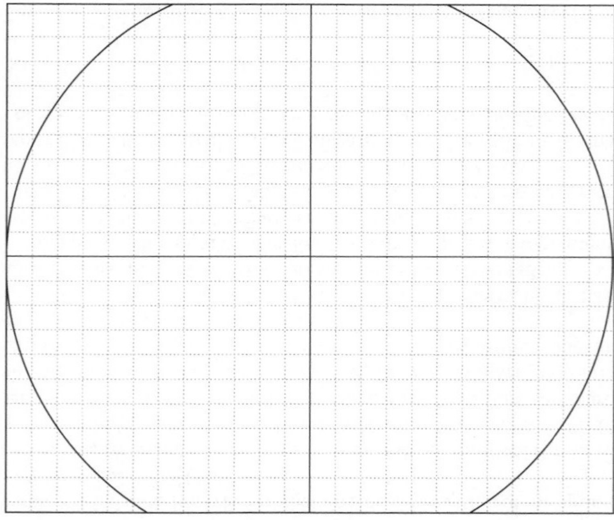

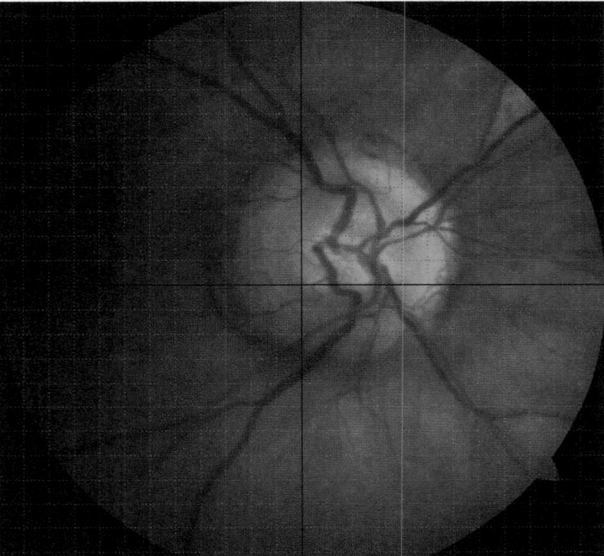

Larger nerve with alpha- and beta-zone parapapillary chorioretinal atrophy.

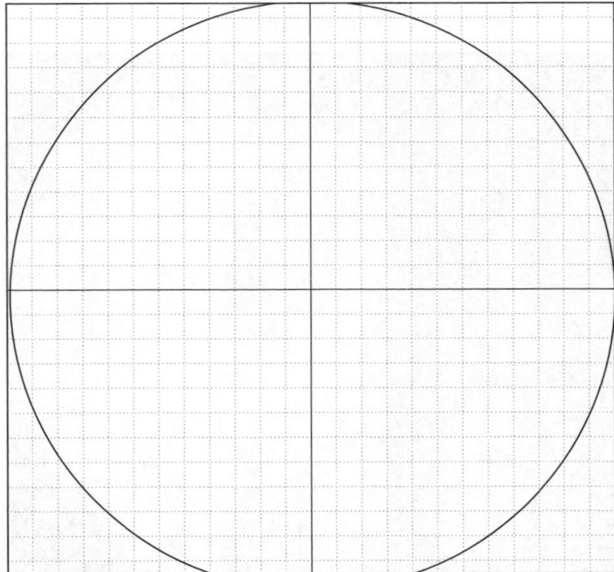

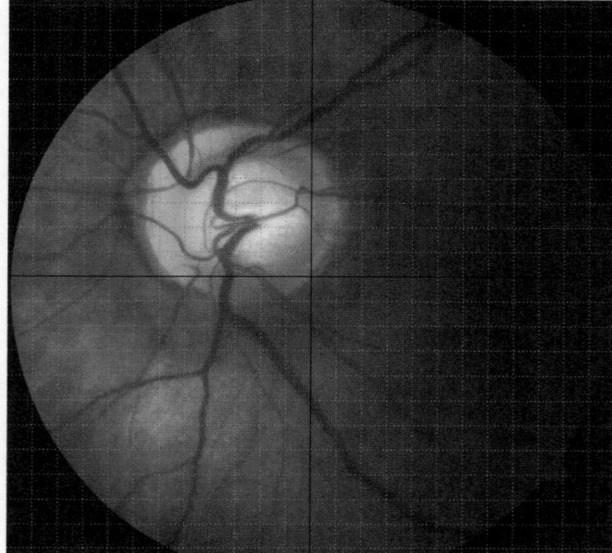

Larger nerve with central retinal vessel trunk nasalization and questionable superior neuroretinal rim thinning.

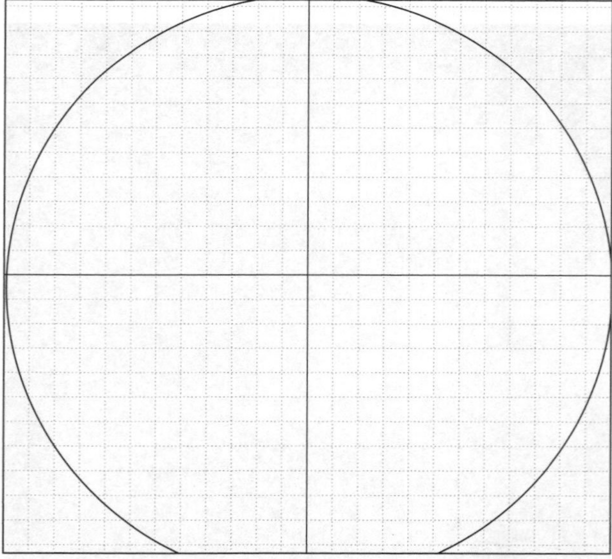

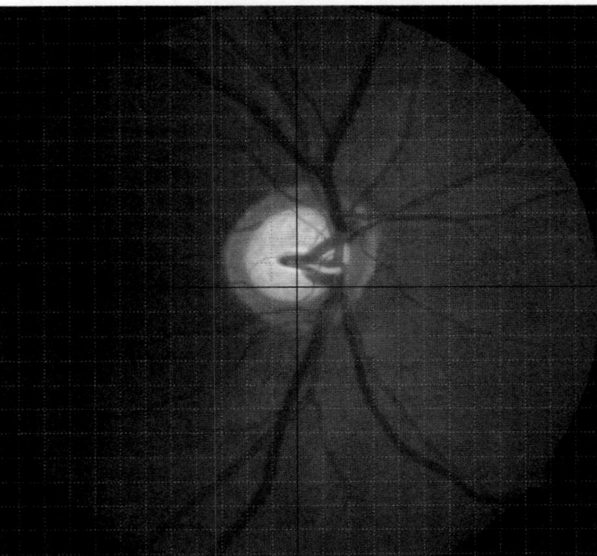

Larger nerve with deeper cup and less visible retinal nerve fiber layer pattern.

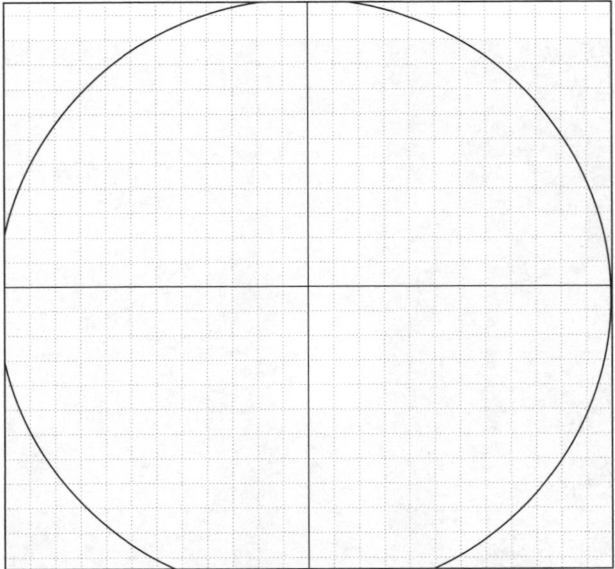

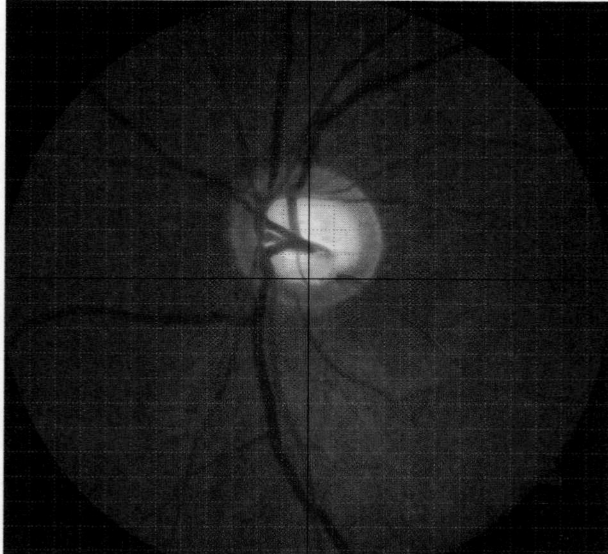

Larger nerve with larger cupping, moderate depth, and suspected inferior retinal arteriole diameter narrowing with correlating inferior rim thinning relative to superior rim width.

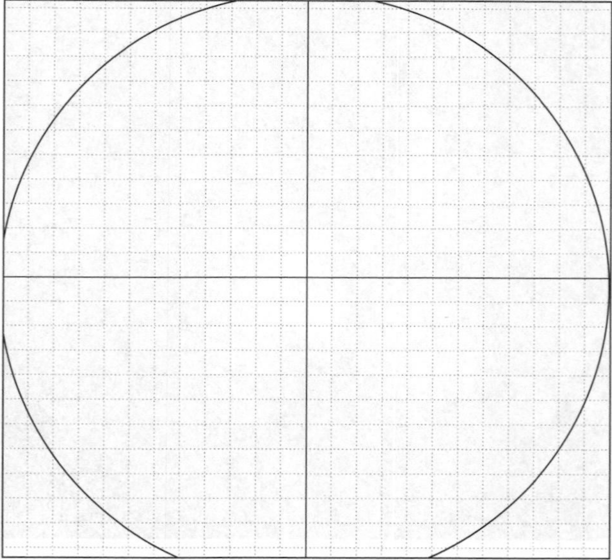

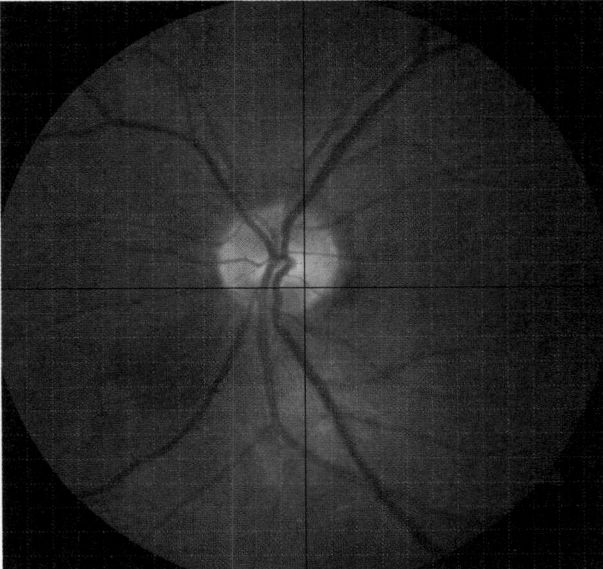

Average-small size nerve with smaller cupping.

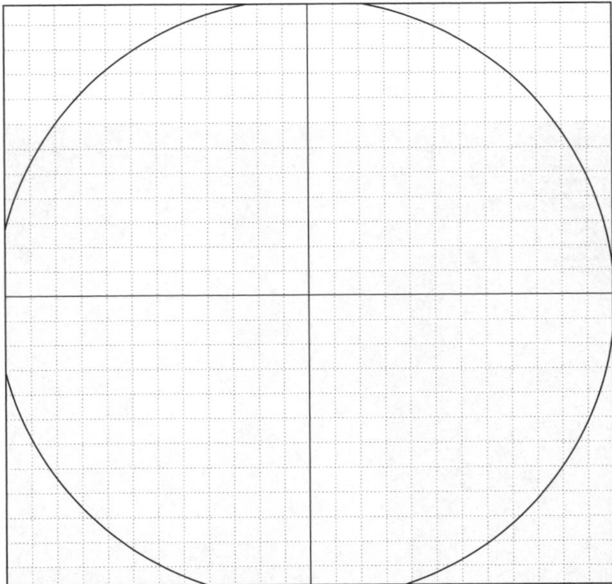

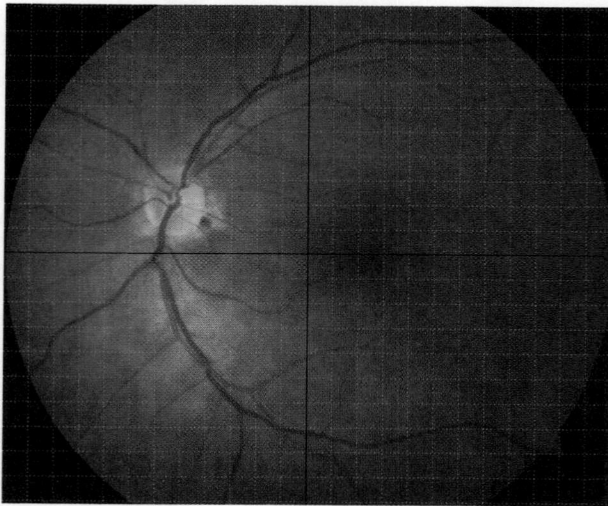

Small, oval-shaped nerve with small cupping.

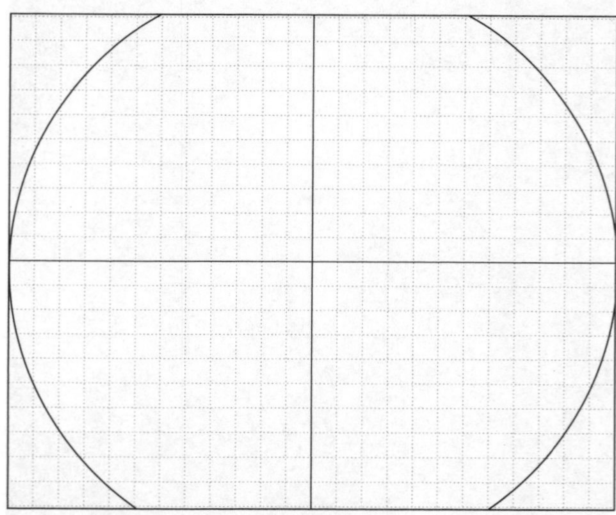

3. OPTIC DISC SHAPE

Overview

The normal shape of the optic disc is slightly vertically oval.[1]

Pearls

- **Vertical disc diameter is about 7%–10% larger than the horizontal disc diameter.**
  - Maximal disc diameter is nearly equal to vertical diameter; horizontal diameter is almost equal to the minimal diameter.
- **Glaucoma susceptibility is mostly *independent* of the shape of the optic disc.**
  - *As a single variable,* optic disc shape is not markedly important for diagnosis and pathogenesis of glaucoma in eyes with myopia <−8 D.
    - However, optic disc shape may affect the distance between the neuroretinal rim and the central retinal vessel trunk location on the lamina cribrosa surface (see Chapter 7).
    - Family history may play a role in optic disc shape.[2]
- **Disc shape is not correlated with age, sex, right eye, left eye, body weight, body height.**
  - High myopia (>−12 D)
    - Disc is more oval, elongated than any *other* group.
    - More obliquely oriented than any other group.
- **Disc shape is correlated with increased corneal astigmatism and amblyopia.**
  - Corneal astigmatism is significantly higher in eyes with tilted discs and significantly lower in eyes with more circular disc shapes.
  - The orientation of the longest disc diameter can indicate the axis of the corneal astigmatism.
    - Consider keratometry and retinoscopy in children if the optic nerve is abnormal in shape.
      - Amblyopia is significantly associated with an elongated optic disc shape and high corneal astigmatism.

References

1. Jonas JB, Budde WM, Panda-Jonas S. Ophthalmoscopic evaluation of the optic nerve head. *Surv Ophthalmol.* 1999;43:293–320.
2. Sanfilippo P, Cardini A, Hewitt A, et al. Optic disc morphology – rethinking shape. *Prog Retin Eye Res.* 2009;28:227–248.

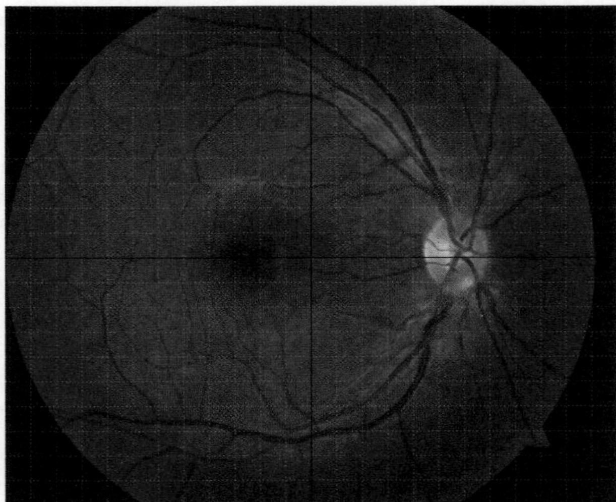

Normal, average-small, oval-shaped nerve with smaller cupping and healthy, robust retinal nerve fiber layer pattern distribution.

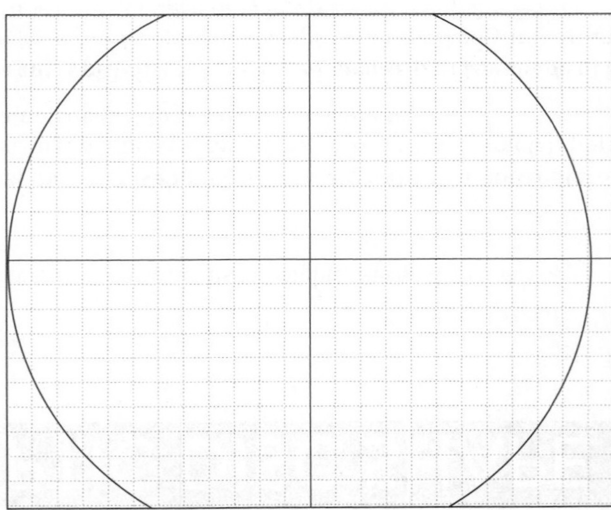

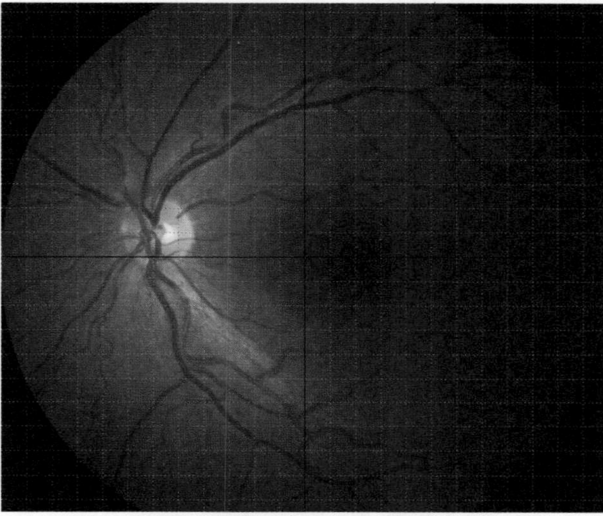

Normal, average-small size nerve with round shape, normal cup shape, and healthy retinal nerve fiber layer pattern distribution.

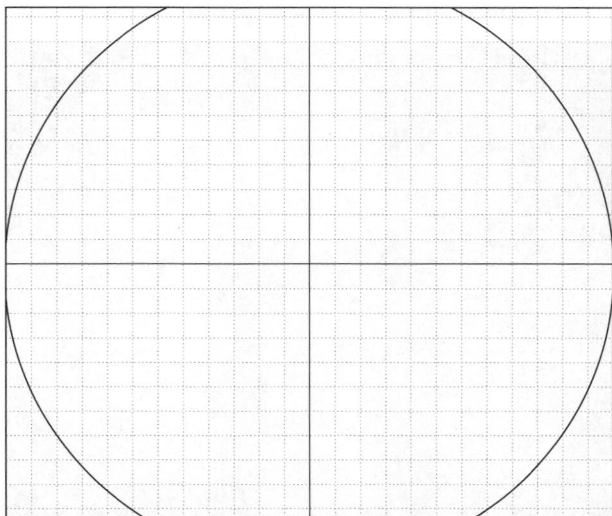

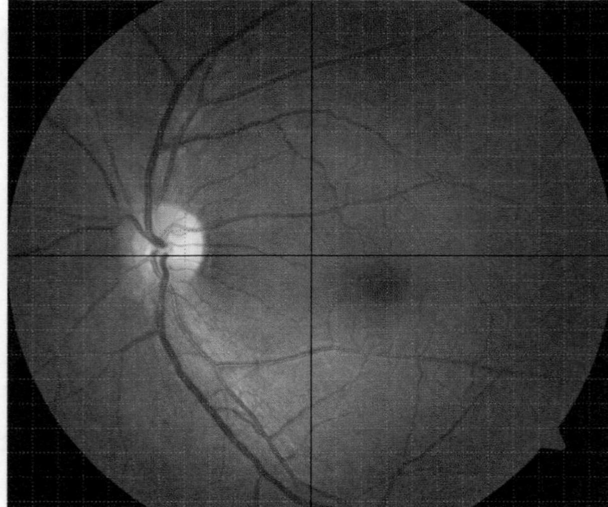

Average-small, oval-shaped nerve with normal size smaller cupping and healthy retinal nerve fiber layer (RNFL) pattern distribution but with questionable temporal pallor. Note: Superior pseudo-RNFL localized defects with an apex that does not extend to the optic nerve and a broad base that does not extend to the horizontal raphe.

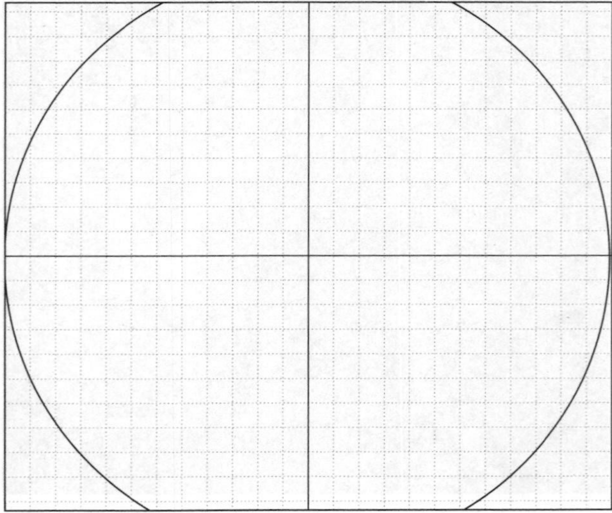

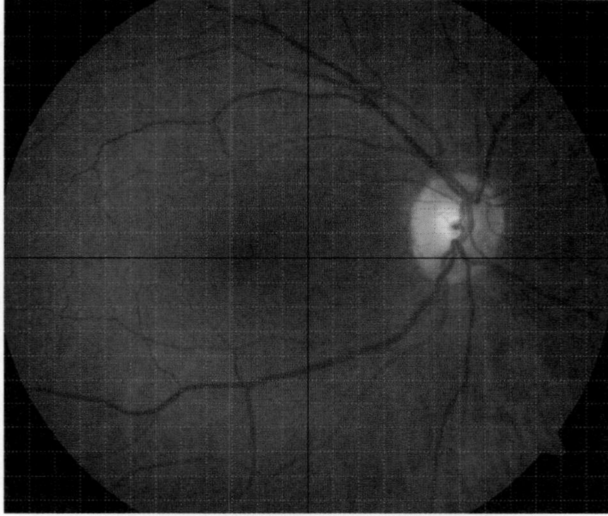

Average size, oval-shaped nerve with vertical cup-to-disc ratio (CDR) greater than the horizontal CDR and suspected superior neuroretinal rim thinning.

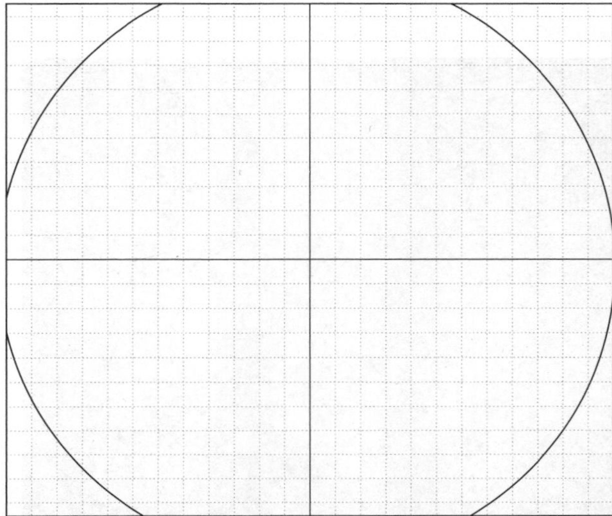

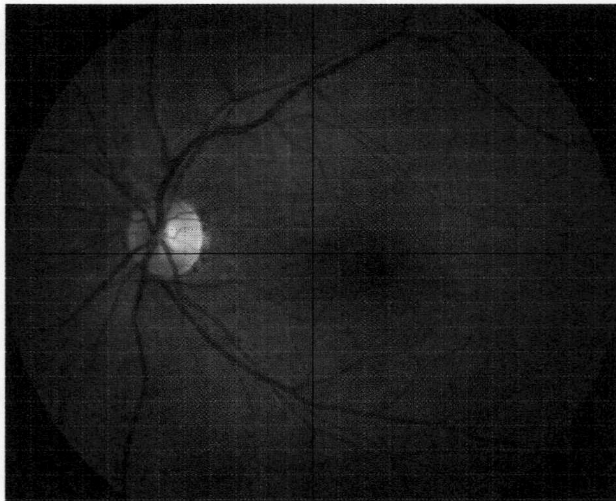

Average size, oval-shaped nerve. Note: Suspected focal temporal pallor.

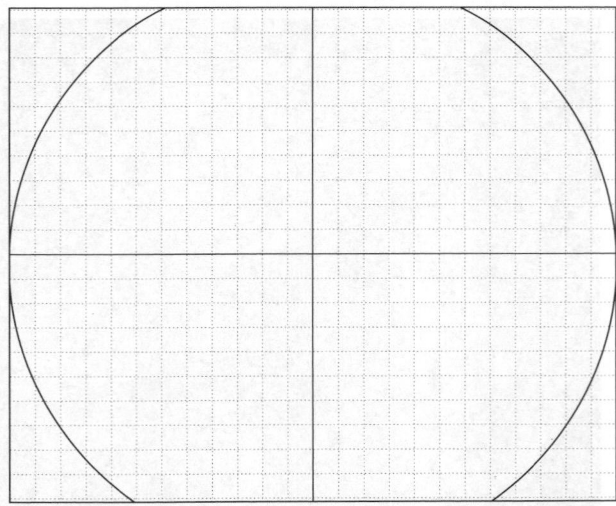

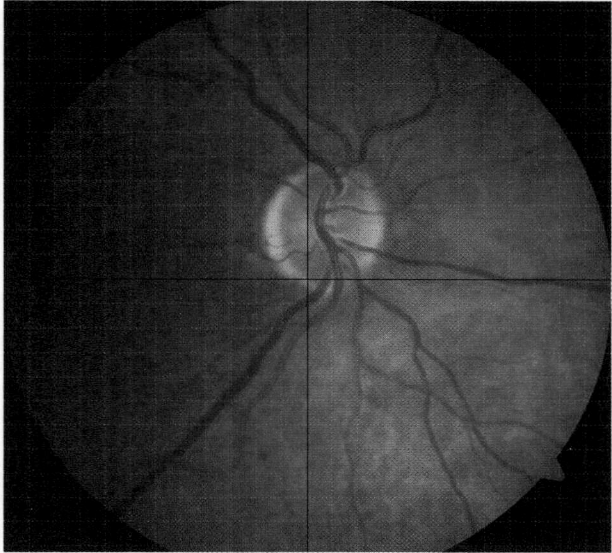

Average size, oval-shaped nerve with minimal cupping.

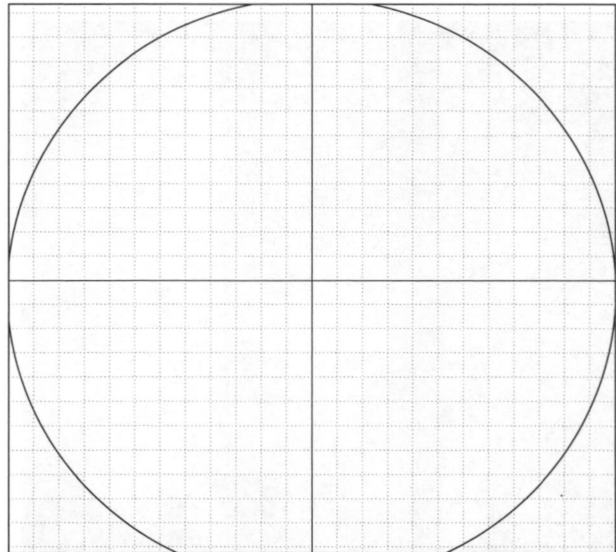

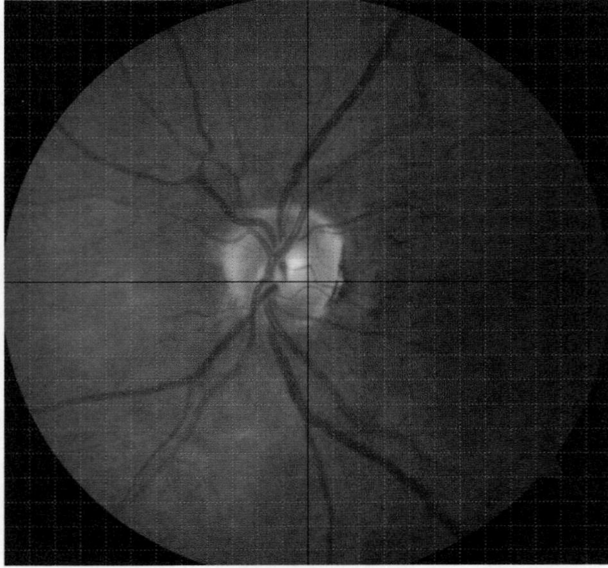

Average size, oval-shaped nerve with normal cupping and healthy neuroretinal rim width.

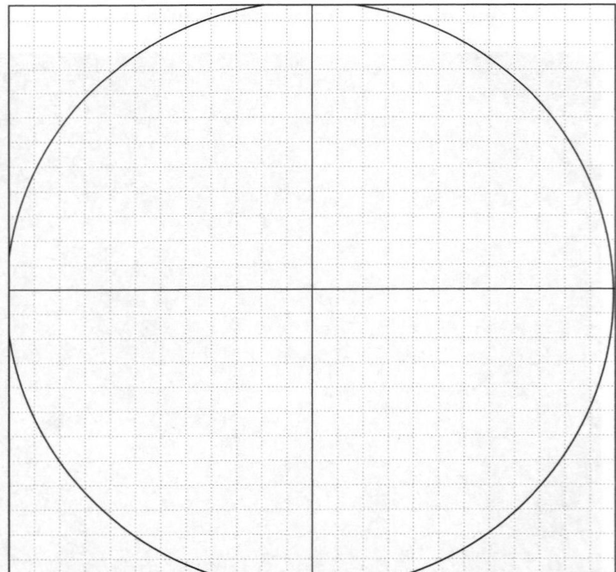

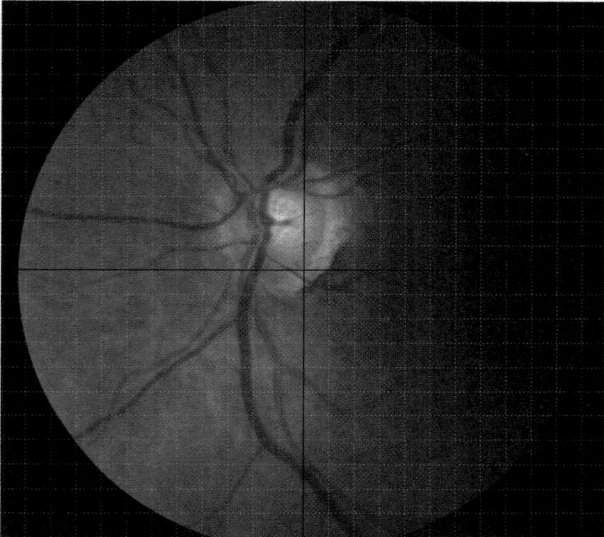

Average-large size, oval-shaped nerve with inferior rim sloping and questionable pallor that extends beyond the cupping.

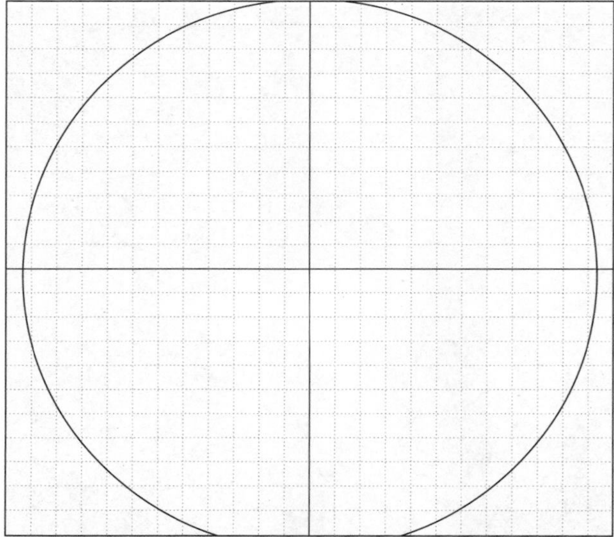

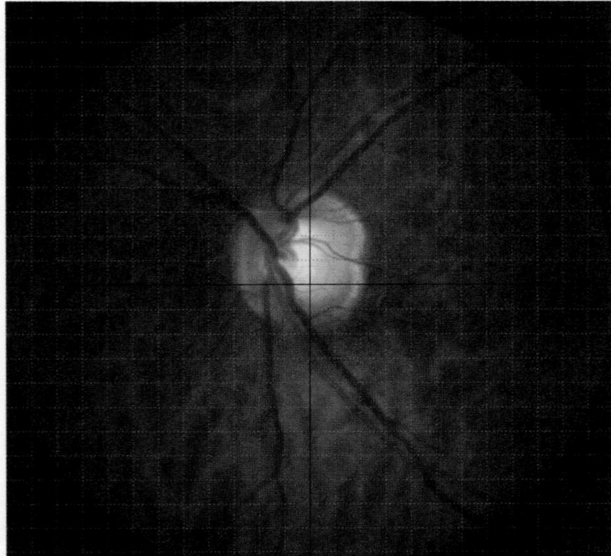

Average size, oval-shaped nerve with questionable inferior vessel baring and relative inferior retinal arteriole diameter narrowing.

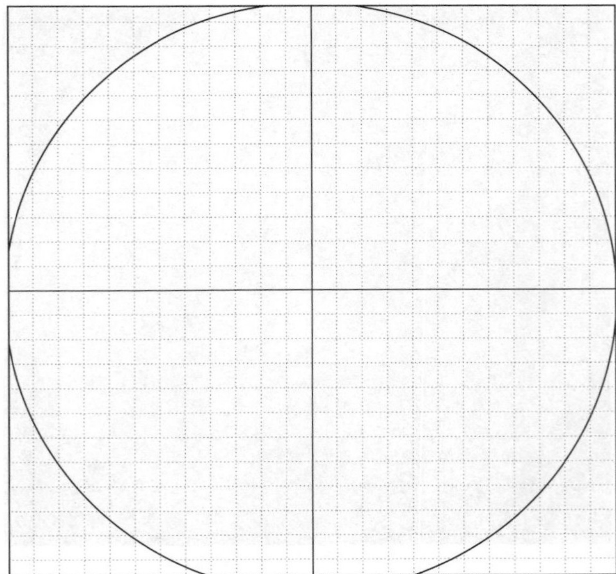

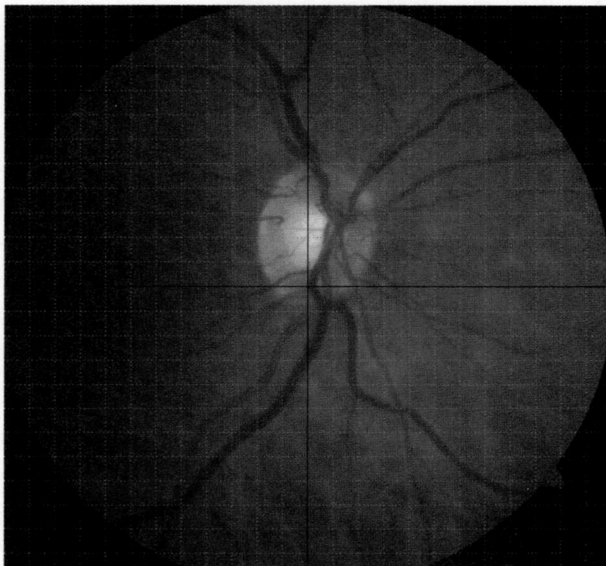

Normal, average size, oval-shaped nerve.

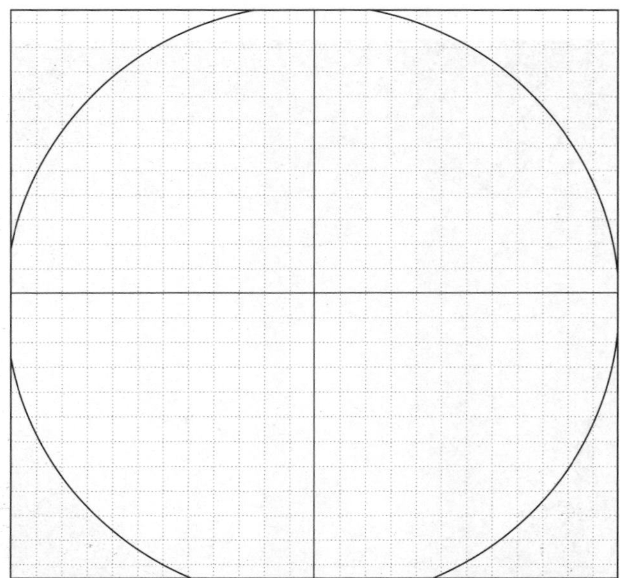

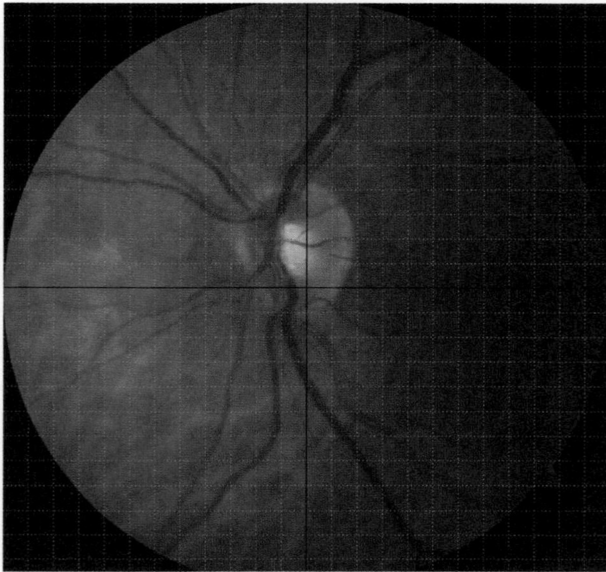

Normal, average size, oval-shaped nerve.

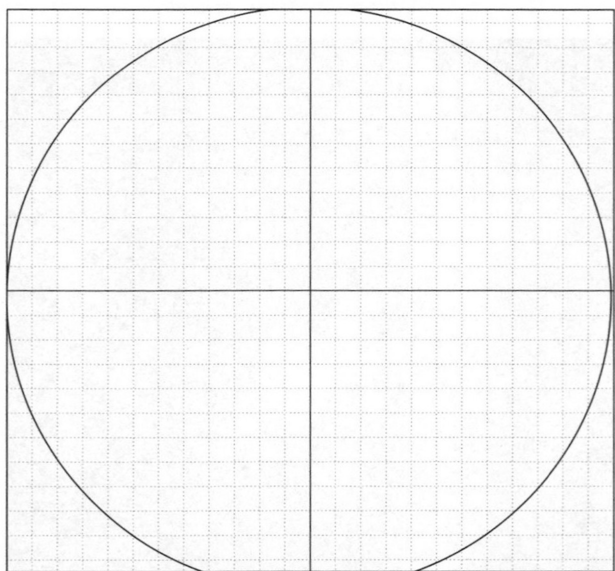

4. OPTIC CUP SHAPE AND DEPTH

Overview

The normal shape of the optic disc is slightly vertically oval, whereas the shape of the optic cup (the excavation in the optic disc) is horizontally oval.[1] Therefore, the *normal* neuroretinal rim is broadest in the inferior and superior disc regions.

Pearls

- **Optic cup shape:**
  - Normal eyes: the horizontal diameter of the optic cup is about 8% greater than the vertical diameter in over 93% of normal eyes.[1]
    - The horizontal optic cup-disc ratio (CDR) is greater than the vertical CDR in *most* normal eyes (i.e., the quotient of the horizontal to vertical CDR is *usually higher* than 1.0).
      - In early to moderate stages of glaucoma, the vertical CDR increases faster than the horizontal CDR, leading to a decrease in the quotient of horizontal to vertical CDR to values *lower* than 1.0.

- **Optic cup depth:**
  - Normal eyes: cup depth is somewhat proportional to the cup area (i.e., the larger the optic cup, the deeper the cup).
  - Glaucoma eyes:
    - Cup depth deepens, depending on the type of glaucoma and level of intraocular pressure (IOP).
      - The optic cup depth is usually greatest in glaucomatous eyes with elevated intraocular pressures.
        - The maximum cup depth, as well as the cup area, cup volume, and CDR area is greater in glaucomatous eyes than nonglaucomatous eyes in large- and average-size optic nerves.[2,3]
      - The optic cup is usually most shallow in glaucomatous eyes with high myopia and senile atrophic morphologic changes.
        - Shallow, diffuse cupping that extends to the disc margin ("saucerization") is an early indicator of glaucoma.

- The depth of the cup may be inversely proportional to the area of parapapillary atrophy.
    - The deeper and steeper the cups, the smaller the area of parapapillary atrophy.

References

1. Jonas JB, Budde WM, Panda-Jonas S. Ophthalmoscopic evaluation of the optic nerve head. *Surv Ophthalmol.* 1999;43:293–320.
2. Medeiros FA, Vizzeri G, Zangwill LM, et al. Comparison of retinal nerve fiber layer and optic disc imaging for diagnosing glaucoma in patients suspected of having the disease. *Ophthalmology.* 2008;115:1340–1346.
3. Okimoto S, Yamashita K, Shibata T, et al. Morphological features and important parameters of large optic discs for diagnosing glaucoma. *PLoS ONE.* 2015;10(3).

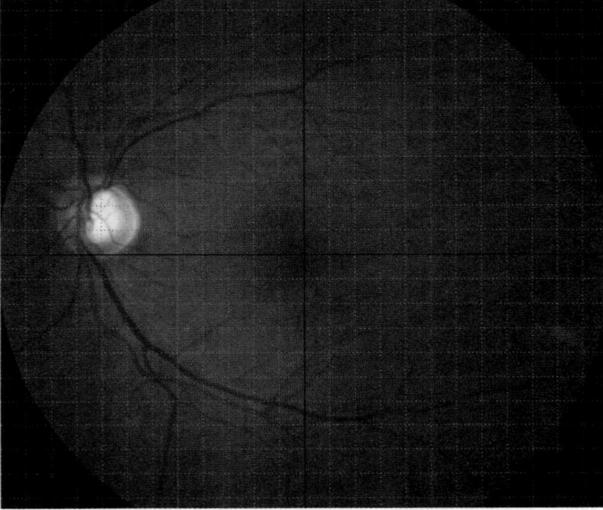

Average size nerve with superior rim thinning and associated relative superior retinal nerve fiber layer (RNFL) loss. Note: Compare to inferior rim with somewhat detectable RNFL pattern and relatively minimal inferior rim thinning.

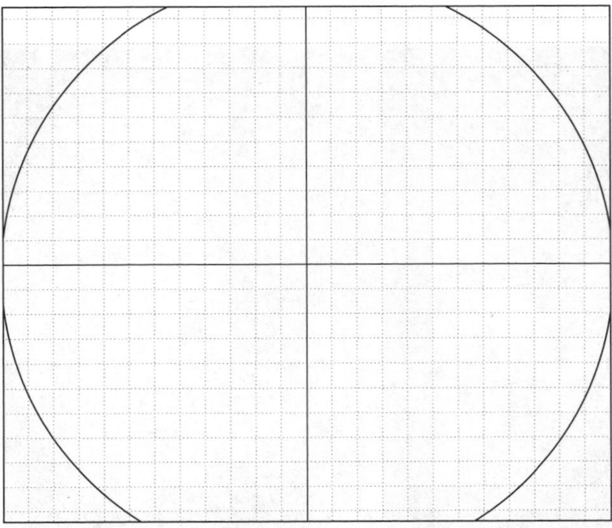

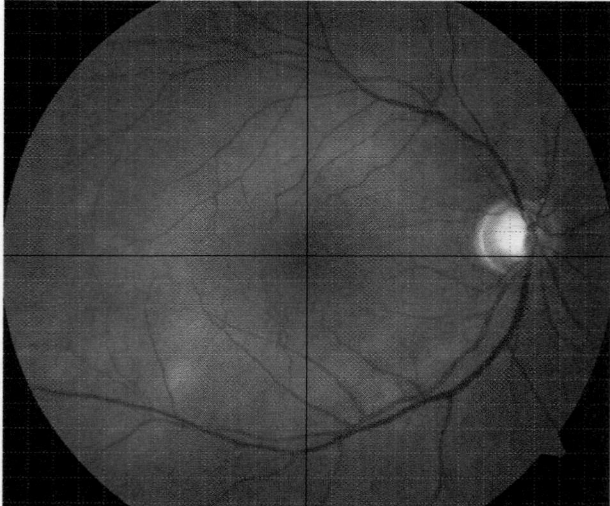

Average size nerve with superior rim thinning and associated relative superior retinal nerve fiber layer (RNFL) loss. Note: Compare to inferior rim with detectable RNFL pattern and relatively minimal inferior rim thinning.

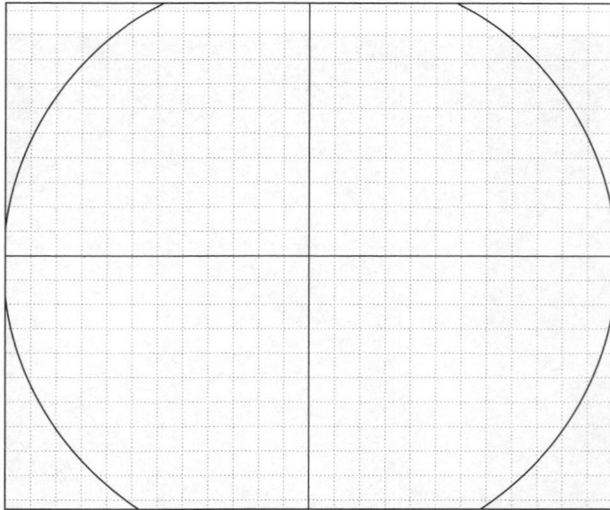

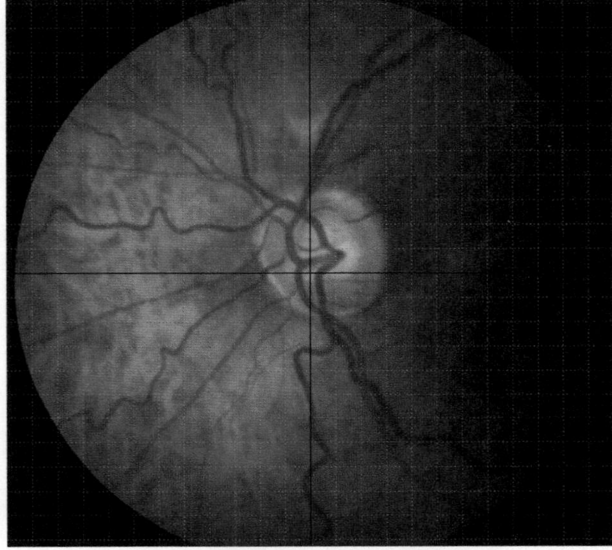

Average size nerve with moderate depth, vertical rim thinning, and correlating retinal arteriole diameter narrowing.

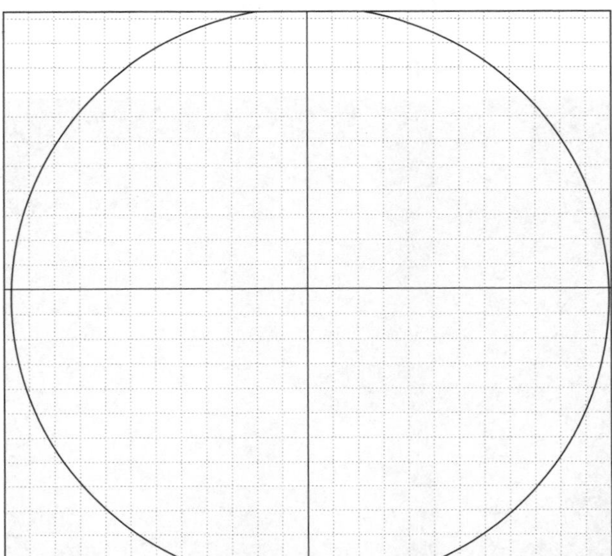

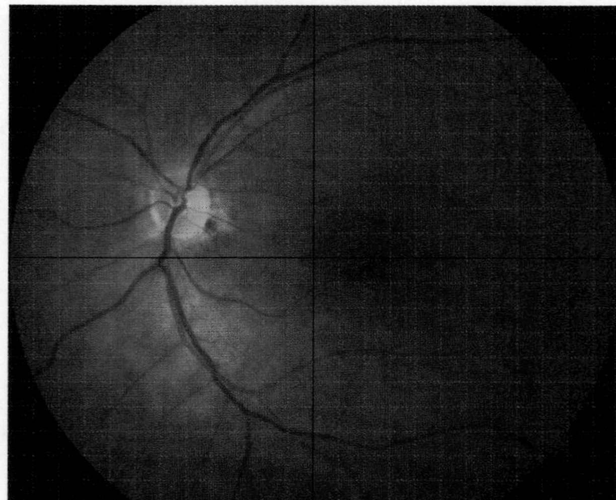

Small nerve, small cupping, shallow depth.

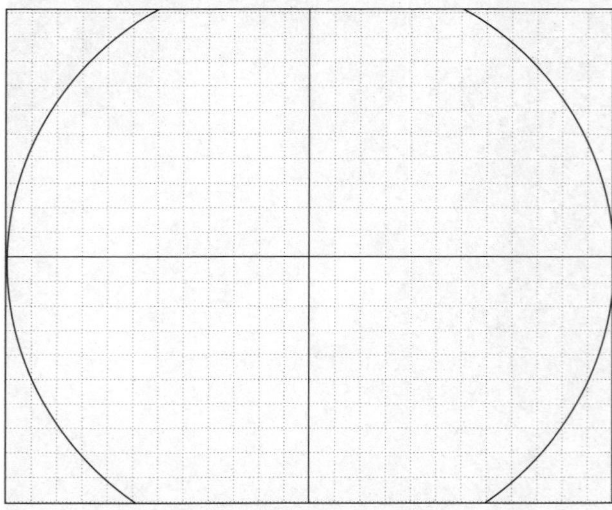

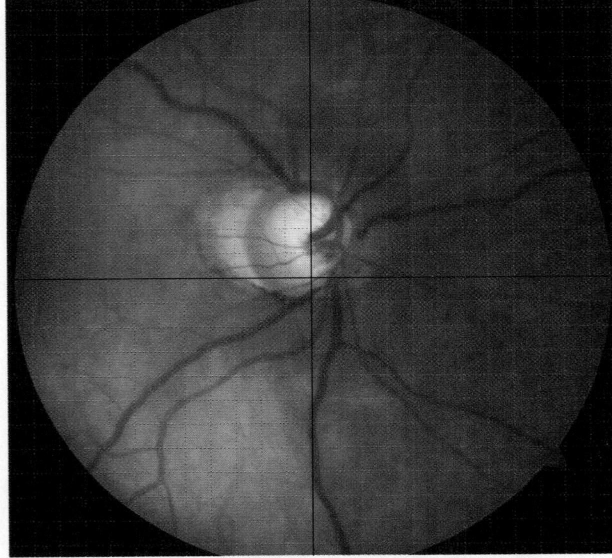

Average size nerve with large, vertical cupping shape and moderate depth.

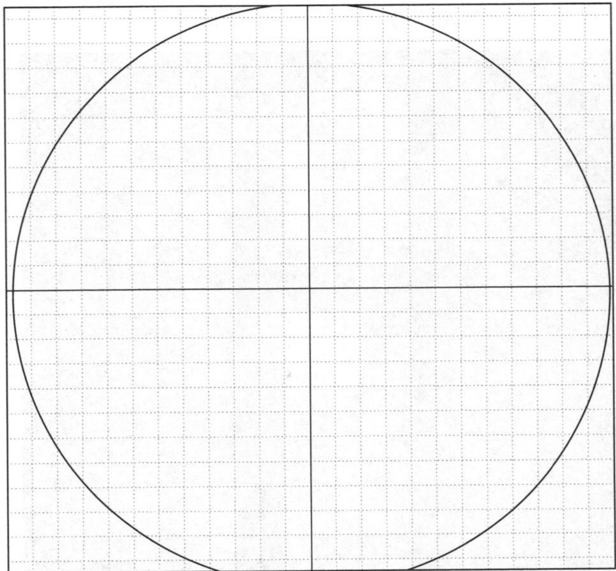

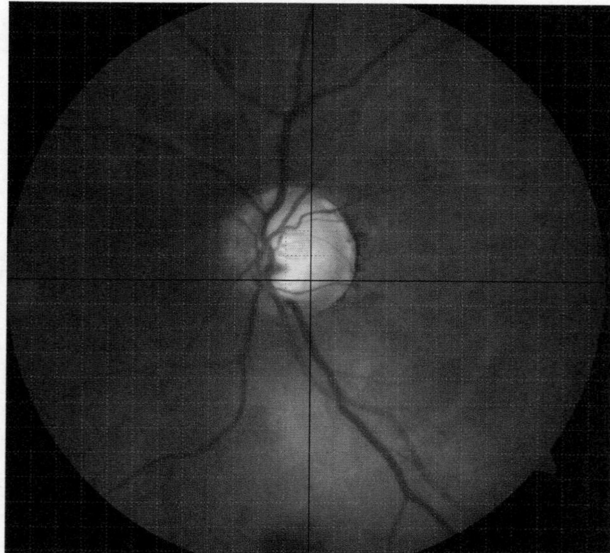

Average size nerve with large, vertical cupping shape and moderate depth.

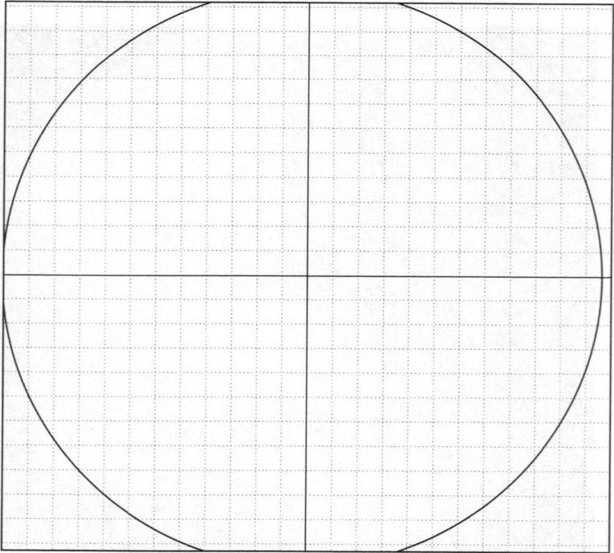

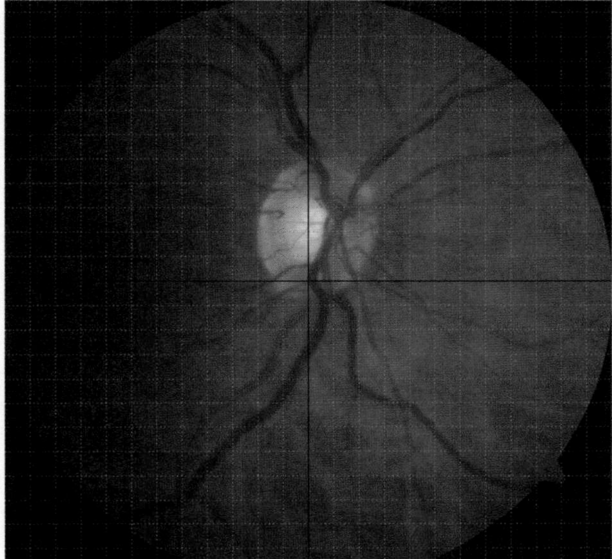

Average size, oval-shaped nerve with oval, shallow cupping.

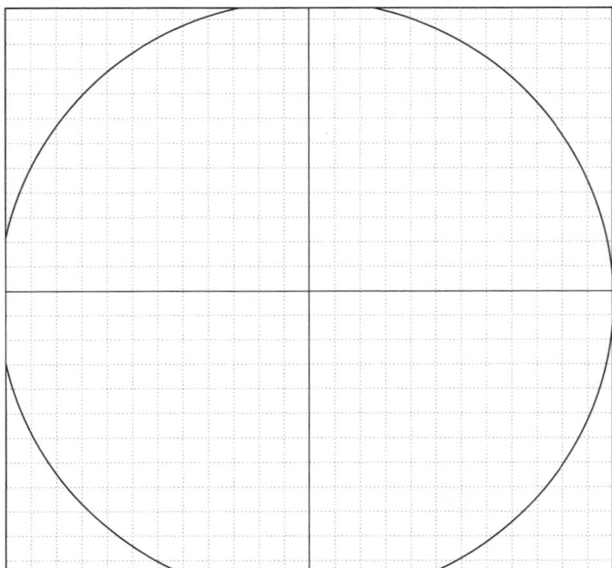

5. OPTIC CUP SIZE IN RELATION TO THE OPTIC DISC SIZE

Overview

Always consider the size of the optic disc when evaluating the size of the optic cup.[1]

Pearls

- **Optic cup size or border is determined by contour and NOT by color.**
  - Must be examined stereoscopically.
  - Similar to optic disc size and neuroretinal rim area, there is considerable normal interindividual optic cup size variability.
    - The size of the optic cup is proportional to the size of the optic disc.
      - The cup- disc ratio (CDR) can range from 0.0 to 0.9 in the normal population with significant overlap between normal patients and glaucomatous patients.[2]
        - Small CDR in smaller nerves, large CDR in larger nerves—both normal.
          - The larger the optic disc, the larger the optic cup.
        - Caution with overdiagnosing large CDRs in large discs.
          - A large optic cup in a large optic disc *should not* automatically be diagnosed as glaucomatous, especially if the other optic nerve features (i.e., neuroretinal rim shape, retinal nerve fiber layer, etc.) are normal.
            - Risk for overtreatment.
        - Caution with underdiagnosing/misdiagnosing average CDR in small discs with or without ocular hypertension.
          - Early or moderate glaucomatous optic nerve damage may erroneously be overlooked in small discs because of "pseudo-normal" appearance.
            - Risk for undertreatment.
            - Carefully examine the parapapillary region for decreased retinal nerve fiber layer visibility (diffuse or focal), decreased arteriole diameter (diffuse or focal), and parapapillary chorioretinal atrophy.

- Constant in size after first years of life.
  - Unlike glaucoma, the optic cup does not significantly enlarge and therefore the neuroretinal rim will not significantly decrease.
    - The increase in cup area is an important marker to differentiate between glaucomatous and nonglaucomatous optic nerve damage.
      - The neuroretinal rim does not significantly decrease in eyes with nonglaucomatous optic nerve damage.
- The *size* of the optic cup may be more predictive of future functional progression than the amount of remaining neuroretinal rim.[3]
  - The amount of remaining neuroretinal rim may correlate better with the patient's current level of functional status.

References

1. Jonas JB, Budde WM, Panda-Jonas S. Ophthalmoscopic evaluation of the optic nerve head. *Surv Ophthalmol.* 1999;43:293–320.
2. Jonas JB, Gusek GC, Naumann GO. Optic disc, cup and neuroretinal rim size, configuration and correlations in normal eyes. *Invest Ophthalmol Vis Sci.* 1988;29:1151–1158.
3. Gardiner S, Johnson C, Demirel S. Cup size predicts subsequent functional change in early glaucoma. *Optom Vis Sci.* 2011;88(12):1470–1476.

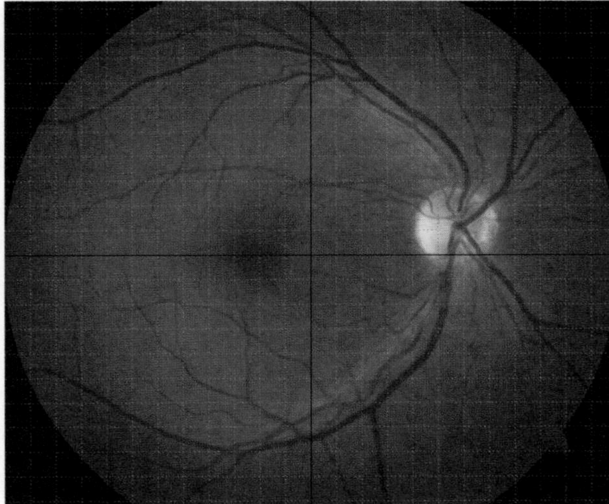

Average-small nerve with minimal cupping and normal, healthy retinal nerve fiber layer appearance.

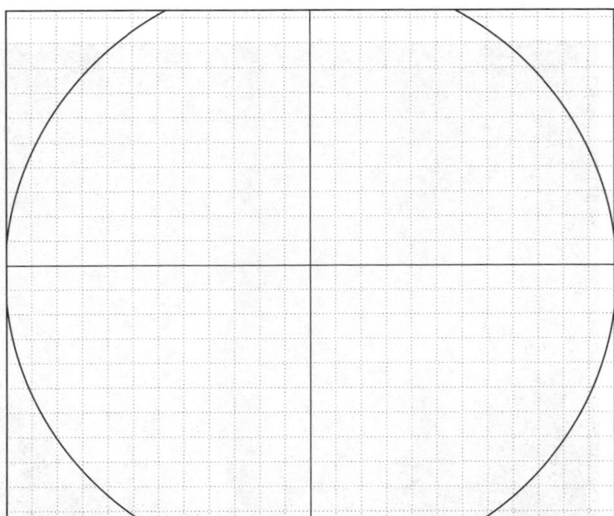

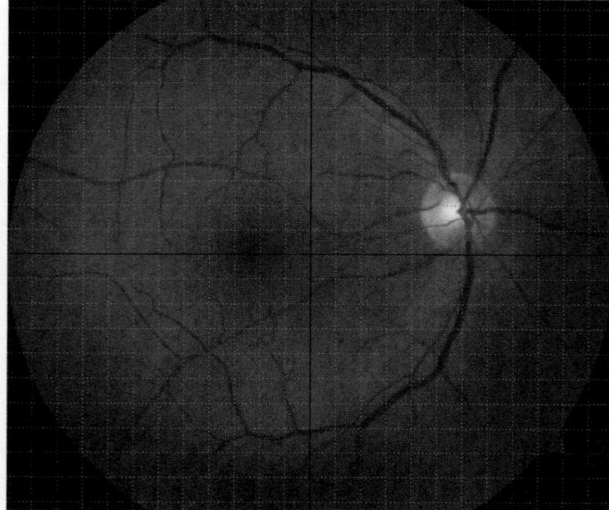

Average-small nerve with normal small cupping and healthy retinal nerve fiber layer appearance.

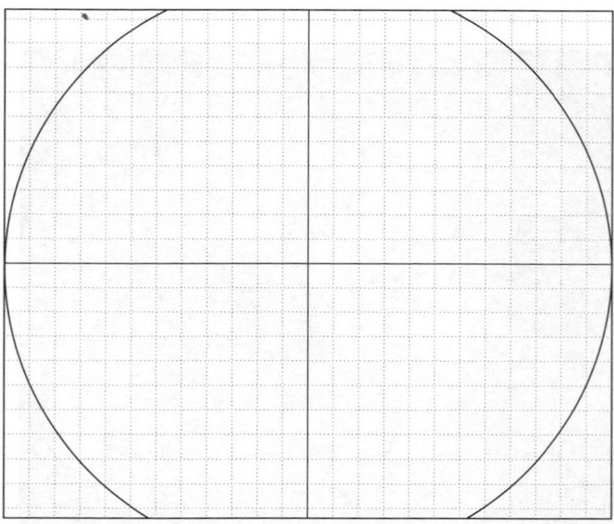

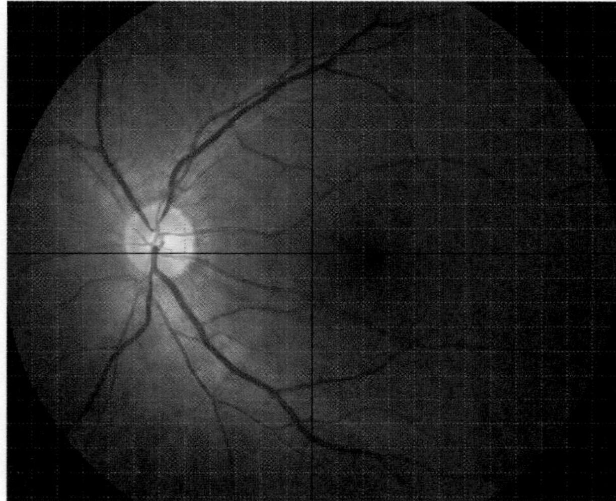

Average-small nerve with minimal cupping and normal, healthy retinal nerve fiber layer appearance.

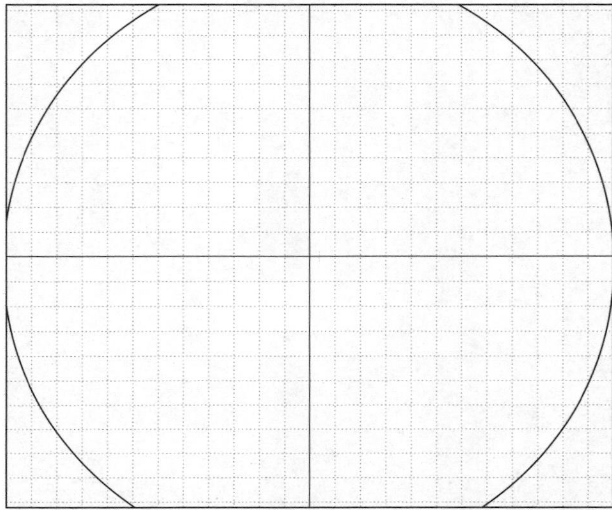

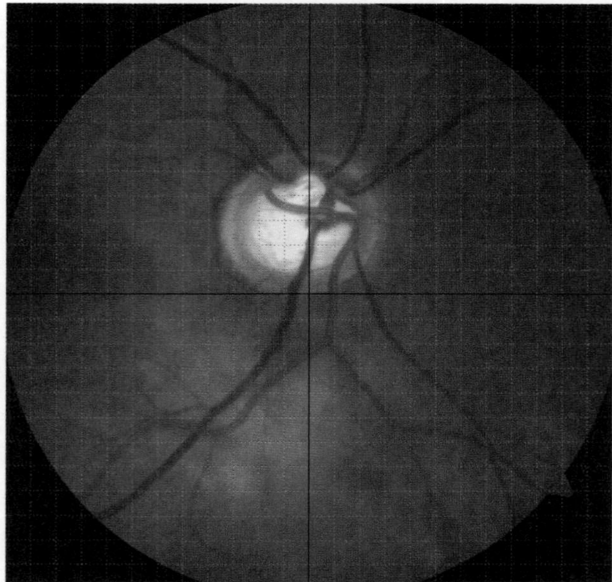

Larger nerve with large "pseudoglaucomatous" cupping, moderate depth, and even rim. All imaging and functional testing for this patient has been, and continues to be, normal. However, these patients are commonly over diagnosed and, as a result, are also overtreated.

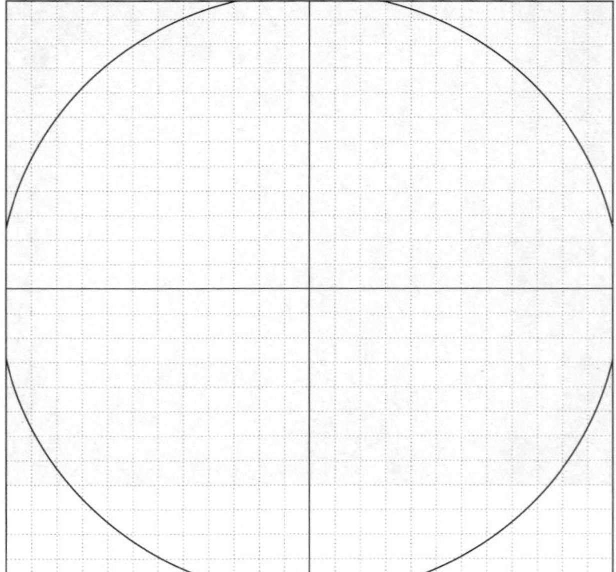

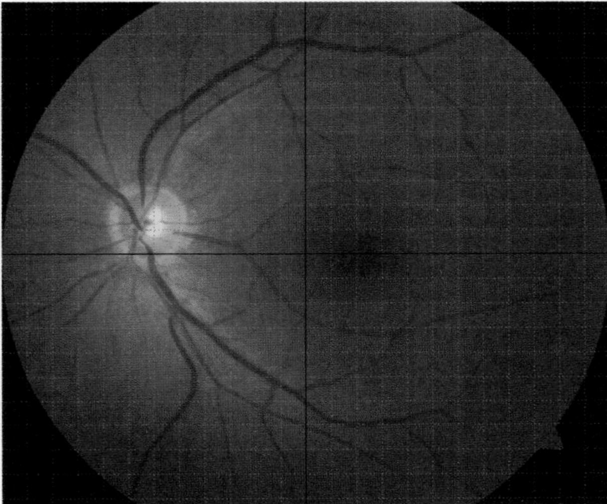

Average-small nerve with average "pseudonormal" cupping, associated superior rim thinning, and correlating early superior-temporal localized retinal nerve fiber layer defect. These patients are commonly underdiagnosed and, as a result, are also undertreated.

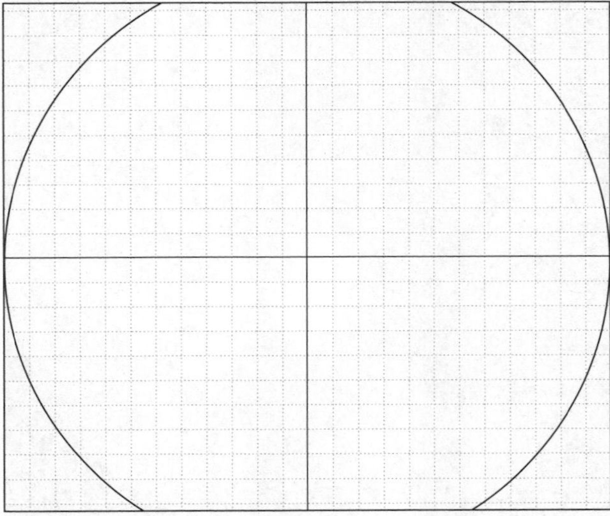

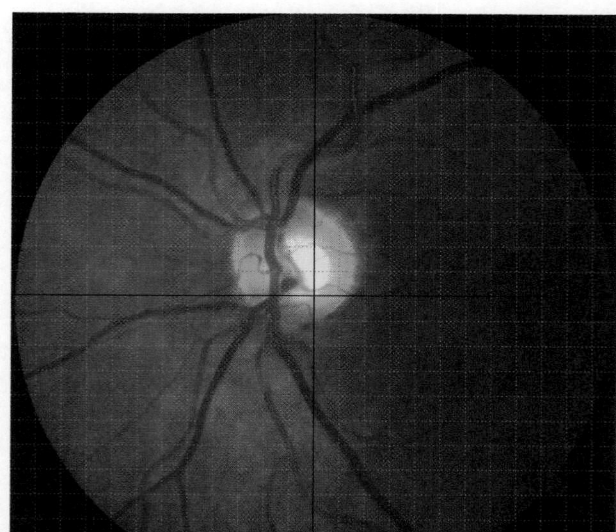

Average size nerve with average-large cupping and suspicious inferior rim thinning.

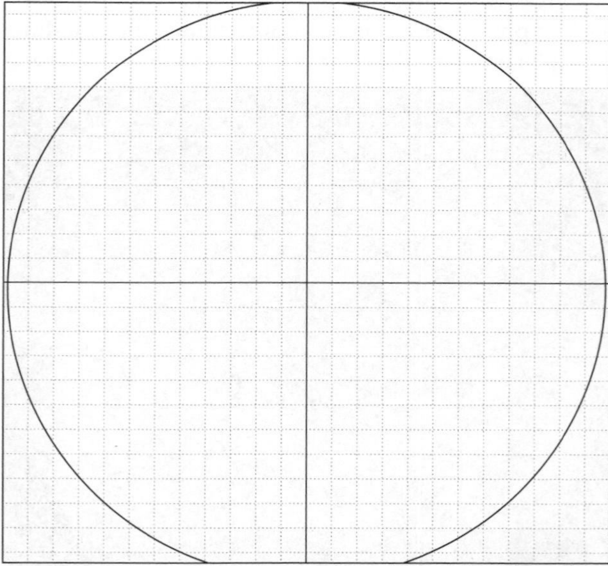

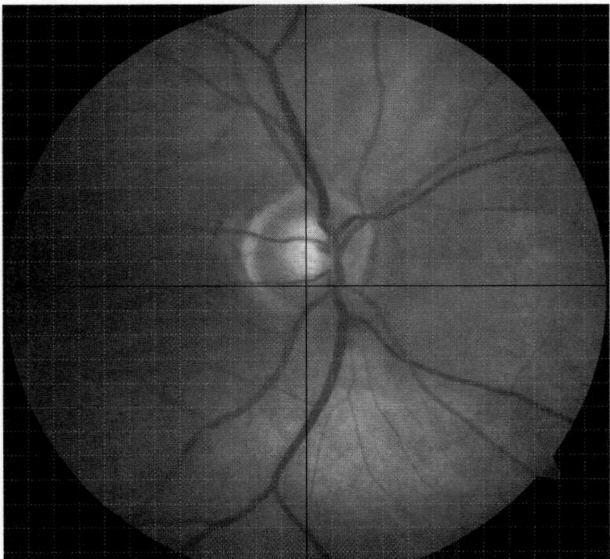

Average size nerve with average-large cupping and suspicious superior rim thinning.

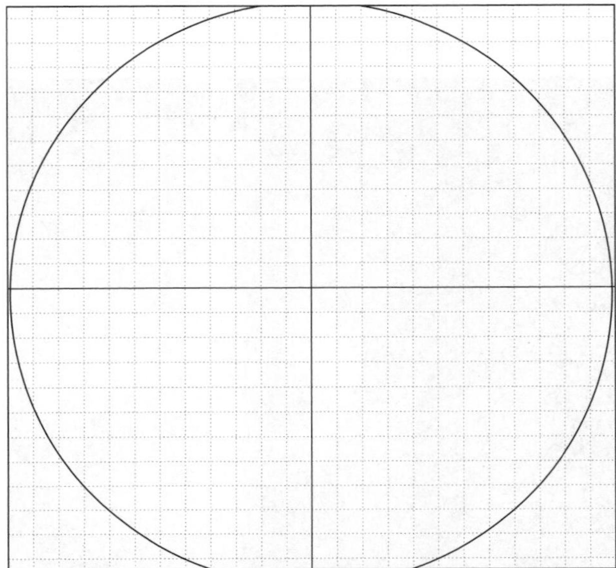

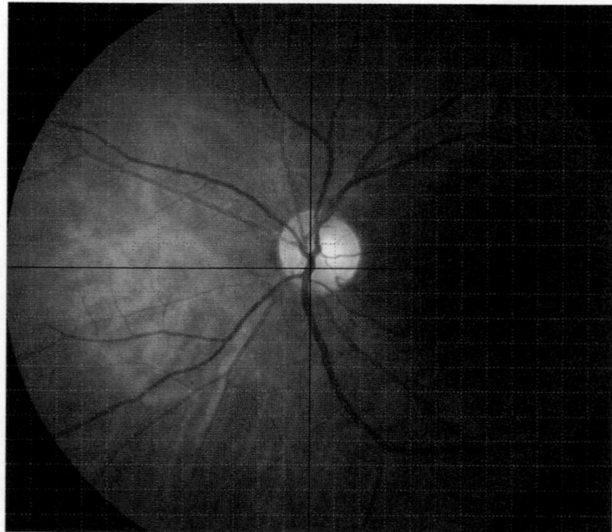

Average size nerve with normal, average size cupping.

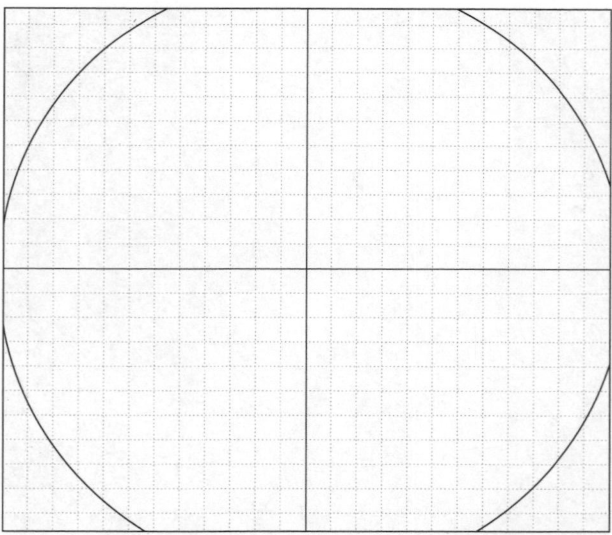

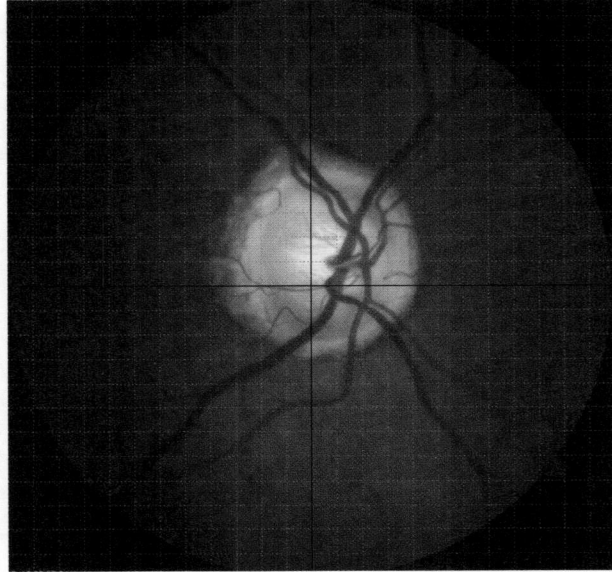

Large nerve with larger cupping and temporal pallor appearance.

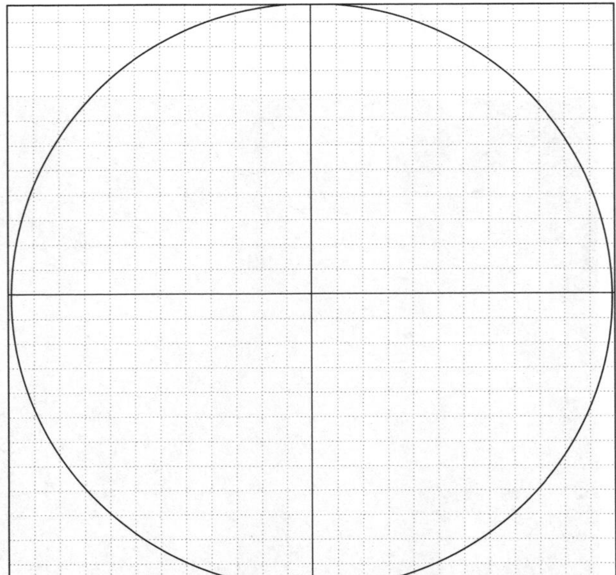

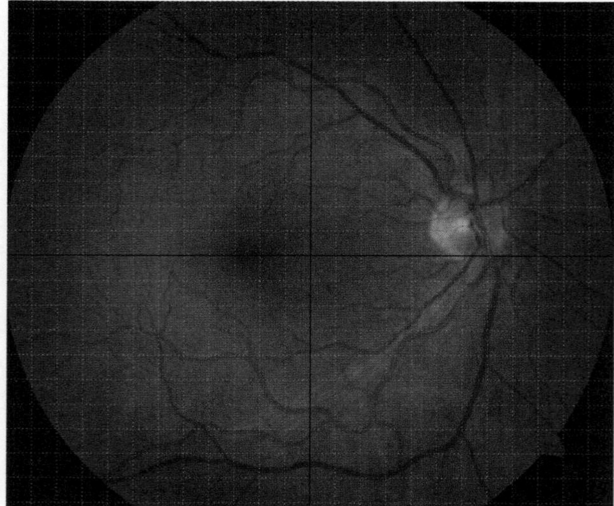

Small nerve with normal, small size cupping.

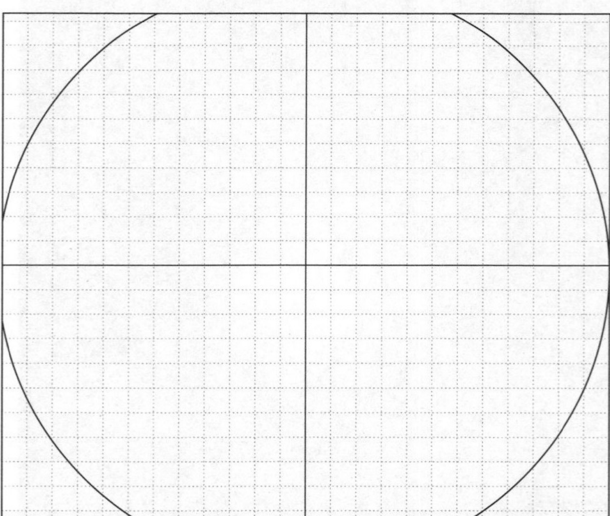

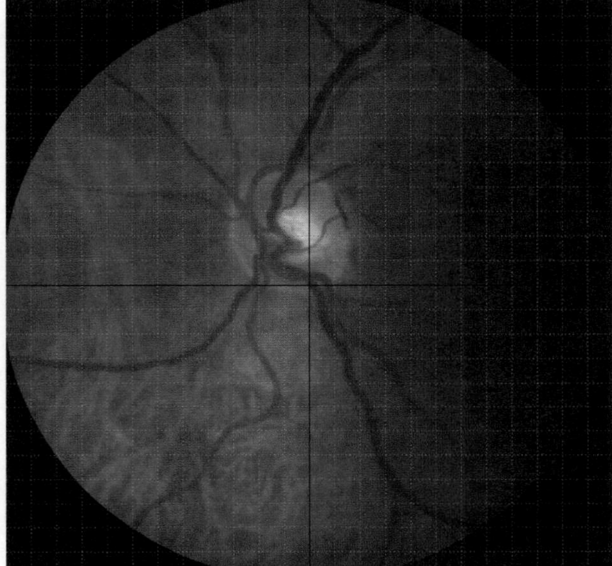

Average size nerve with normal, average size cupping.

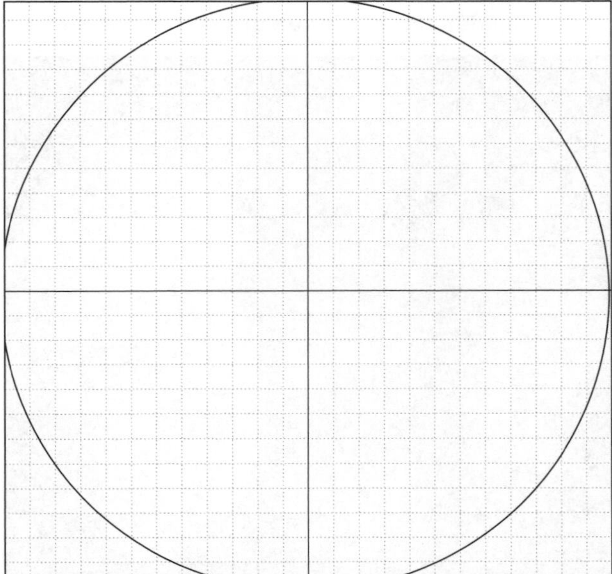

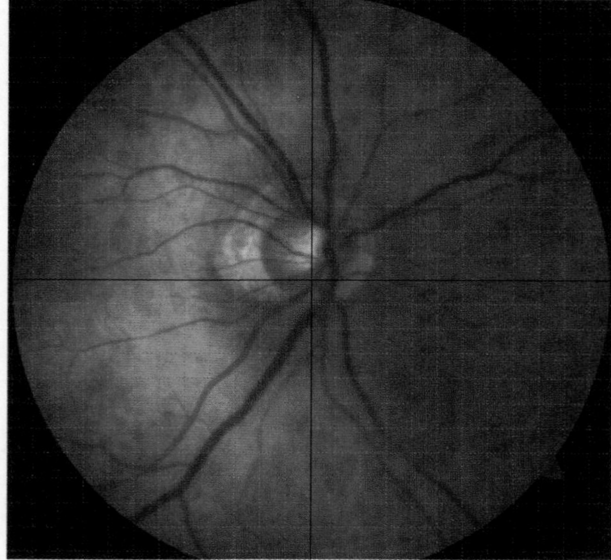

Average size nerve with average-large cupping, suspicious superior-temporal thinning, and superior-temporal parapapillary atrophy.

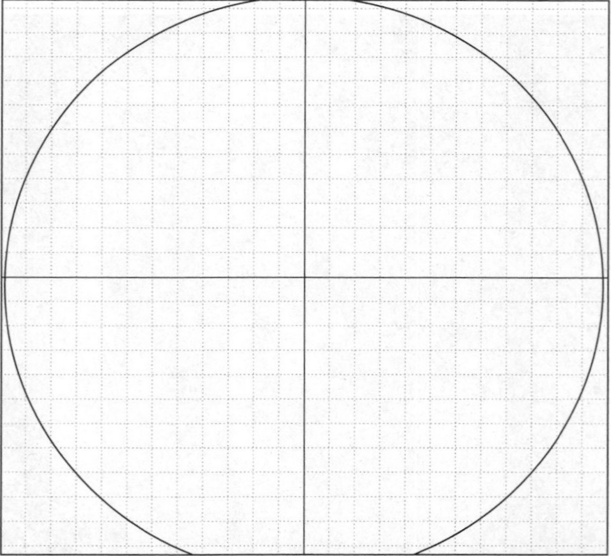

6. NEURORETINAL RIM SIZE, SHAPE, AND PERFUSION

Overview

A careful evaluation of the neuroretinal rim is critical in diagnosing early glaucoma, monitoring for glaucomatous progression, and differentiating between glaucomatous and nonglaucomatous optic neuropathy. In glaucoma, the neuroretinal rim shape is an indicator of the stage of disease and a strong indicator for glaucomatous visual field loss.

Pearls

- **Neuroretinal rim size:**
  - The neuroretinal rim is one of the *most* important variables[1] to accurately diagnose glaucoma earlier and detect progression sooner.
    - Similar to optic disc size and optic cup size, there is high interindividual neuroretinal rim area variability within the normal population and significant overlap between normal eyes and glaucomatous eyes.
      - Neuroretinal rim area is directly proportional to the optic disc area
    - For more accurate diagnosis, divide the optic disc into sectors.
      - There is *preferential loss* of neuroretinal rim in the inferior and superior optic disc regions in the early to moderate stages of the disease.
    - Rim area is *greatest* with no disc cupping; less with temporal flat/sloping of the optic cup, and *least* in eyes with circular, steep disc cupping.
    - Rim area and disc area correspond to optic disc size, optic fiber count, and total area of the lamina cribrosa pores.
    - The nerve fibers within the neuroretinal rim are retinotopically arranged.
      - Axons from ganglion cells close to the optic disc are arranged more centrally in the optic disc, whereas axons from cells in the retinal periphery are located at the optic nerve head margins.

- **Neuroretinal rim shape:**
  - Because of the normal vertical oval shape of optic disc and the normal horizontal oval shape of the optic cup, the neuroretinal rim usually follows "ISNT rule."
    - Inferior neuroretinal rim width is usually most broad, then superior neuroretinal rim, and then nasal neuroretinal rim, with the temporal neuroretinal rim usually being the thinnest sector.
  - Helpful in diagnosing patients with ocular hypertension or early glaucoma prior to visual field defects.
    - Characteristic shape is highly critical in the diagnosis of *early* glaucomatous optic nerve damage in patients with ocular hypertension prior to white-on-white visual field defects.
  - The shape of the neuroretinal rim is positively associated with the following:
    - The diameter of the retinal arterioles: wider in the inferior temporal (IT) arcade than in superior temporal (ST) arcade.
    - The visibility of the retinal nerve fiber layer bundle pattern: usually greatest visibility in the IT sector than the ST sector.
    - The laminar cribrosa morphology: the largest pores, and therefore the least amount of interpore connective tissue, are found in the inferior and superior regions as compared with the temporal and nasal sectors.
- **Glaucomatous neuroretinal rim damage:**
  - The neuroretinal rim commonly shows preferential rim loss, *depending on the stage of the disease:*
    - Early glaucoma: rim loss is usually in the IT and ST sectors.[1–4]
      - Carefully examine these areas for focal neuroretinal rim shape notching.
    - Moderate glaucoma: rim loss is usually in the temporal horizontal sector.
    - Advanced: rim loss is usually in the nasal inferior and then finally in the nasal superior sector.
  - The sequence of preferential neuroretinal sector rim loss (IT → ST→ temporal horizontal → nasal inferior → nasal superior) correlates with the progression of visual field defects:
    - Early visual field loss: superior and inferior (paracentral and/or nasal) visual field defects.
    - Advanced visual field loss: island of remaining visual function in the temporal inferior part of the visual field surrounded by dense depression.
    - The greater the distance from the central retinal vessel trunk location on the lamina cribrosa to the neuroretinal rim, the greater the neuroretinal rim damage and the corresponding visual field defect.
- **Neuroretinal rim pallor**
  - A *common clinical endpoint* of several different nonglaucomatous optic neuropathies and neurologic diseases.
    - *More* noticeable in eyes with nonglaucomatous optic neuropathy than in eyes with glaucoma.

- In glaucoma, if there is pallor, the overall pallor of the optic disc is mainly due to the enlargement of the pale optic cup.

- Nonglaucomatous optic nerve damage is usually not associated with neuroretinal rim loss, just pallor.
  - Pallor extends beyond cupping.
  - Pallor is one of the variables that is helpful to differentiate between glaucomatous and nonglaucomatous optic neuropathy.

References

1. Jonas JB, Budde WM, Panda-Jonas S. Ophthalmoscopic evaluation of the optic nerve head. *Surv Ophthalmol.* 1999;43:293–320.
2. Jonas JB, Gusek GC, Naumann GO. Optic disc, cup and neuroretinal rim size, configuration and correlations in normal eyes. *Invest Ophthalmol Vis Sci.* 1988;29:1151–1158.
3. Hammel N, Belghith A, Zangwill L, et al. Rate and pattern of rim area loss in healthy and progressing glaucoma eyes. *Ophthalmology.* 2016;123(4):760–770.
4. Lloyd M, Mansberger S, Cioffi G, et al. Features of optic disc progression in patients with ocular hypertension and early glaucoma. *J Glaucoma.* 2013;22(5):343–348.

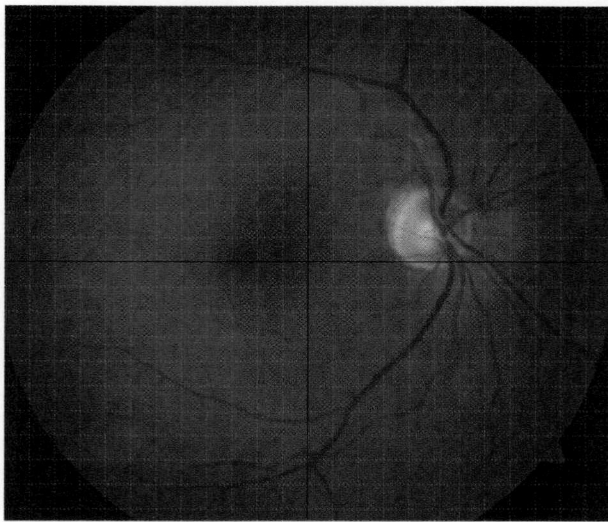

Average size nerve with temporal pallor that extends beyond the cupping.

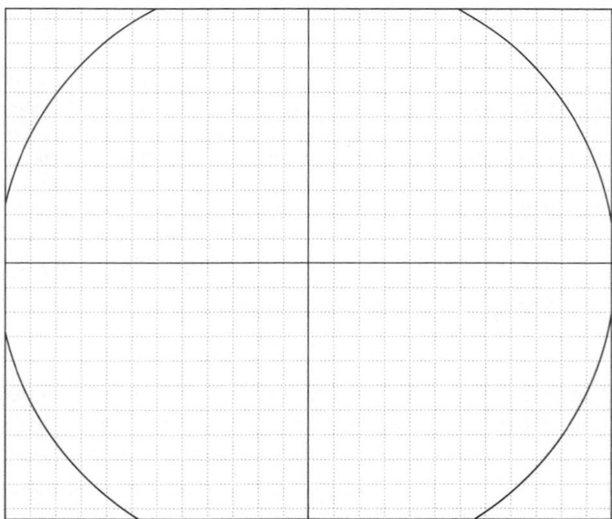

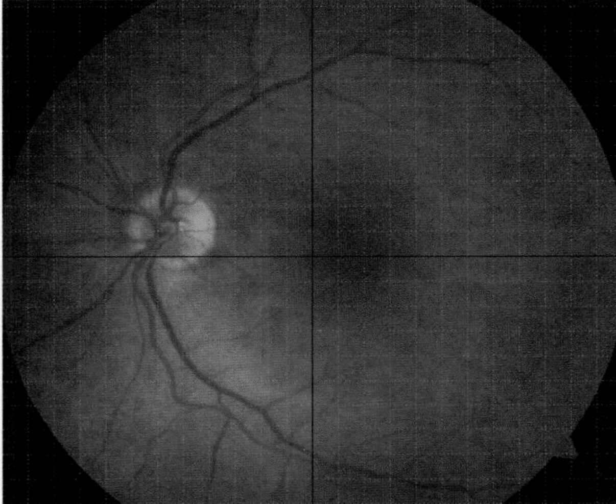

Small nerve with subtle temporal sectoral pallor that extends beyond the small cupping. Interocular and intraocular optic nerve evaluation is helpful in detecting optic nerve pallor.

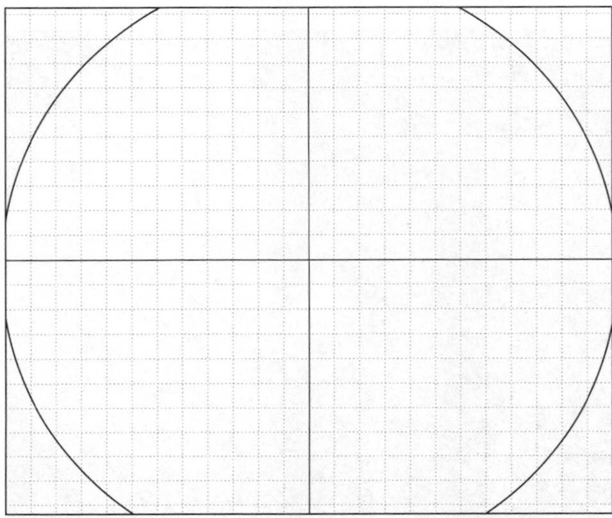

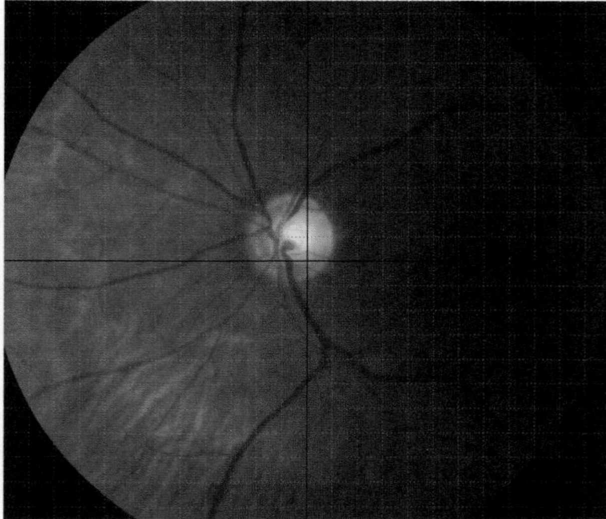

Average size nerve with subtle superior temporal pallor that extends beyond the average cupping. Interocular and intraocular optic nerve evaluation is helpful in detecting optic nerve pallor.

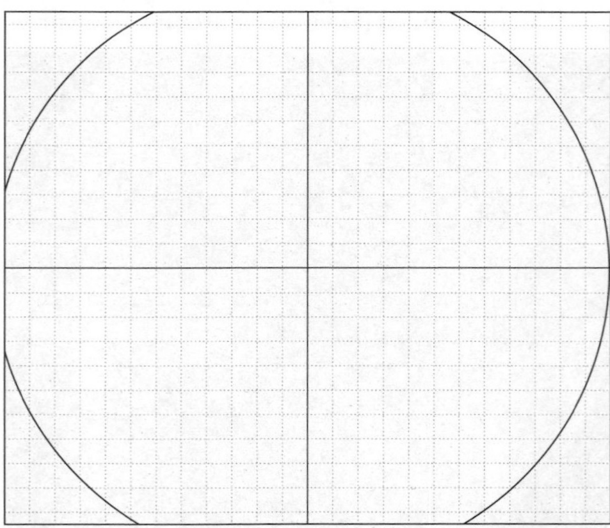

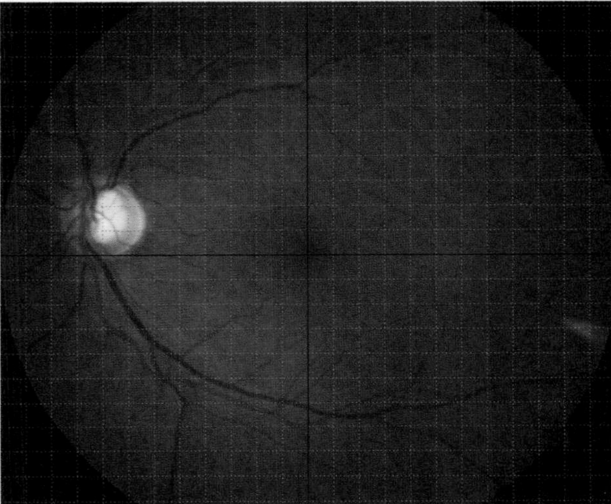

Average size nerve with large cupping, superior rim thinning, and superior retinal nerve fiber layer loss. Note: Normal rim perfusion despite significant cupping.

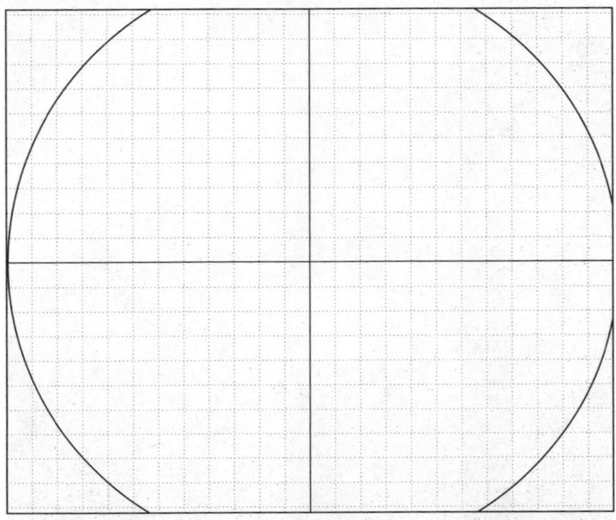

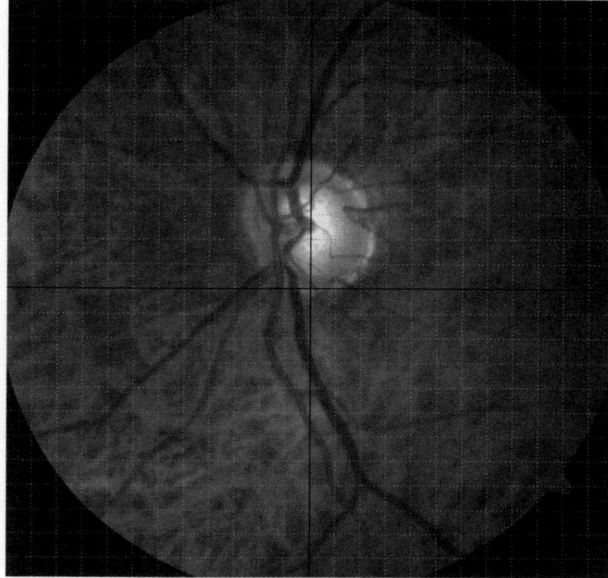

Average size nerve with vertical rim thinning. Note: Normal rim perfusion despite significant cupping.

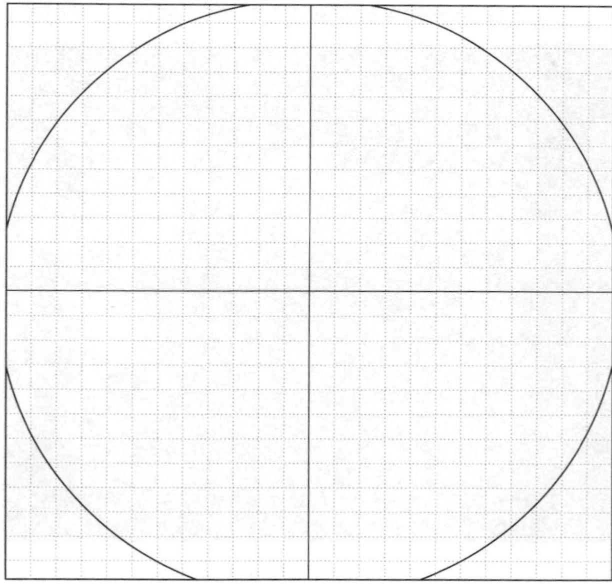

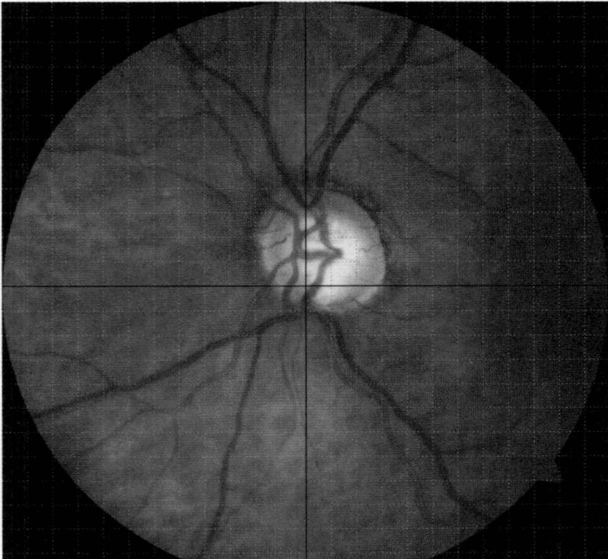

Average size nerve with inferior rim thinning. Note: Normal rim perfusion despite significant cupping.

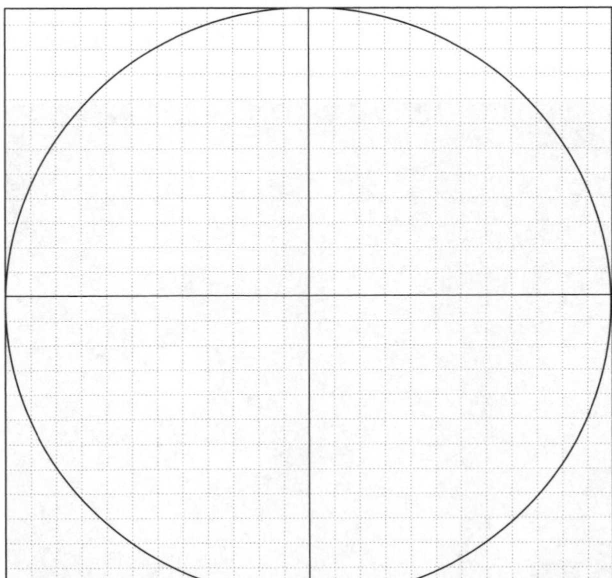

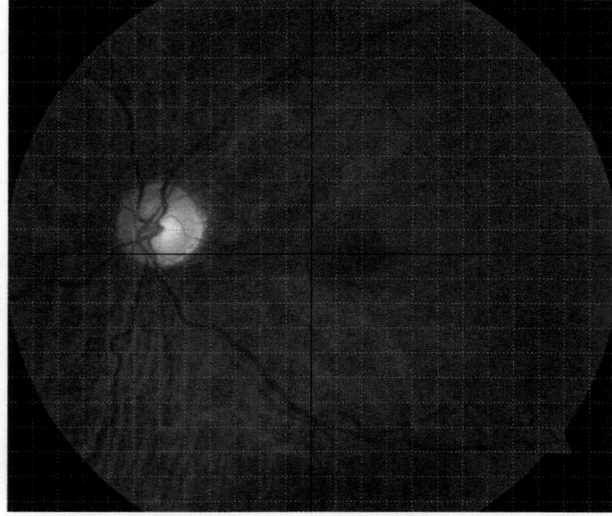

Average size nerve with temporal pallor that extends beyond the cupping.

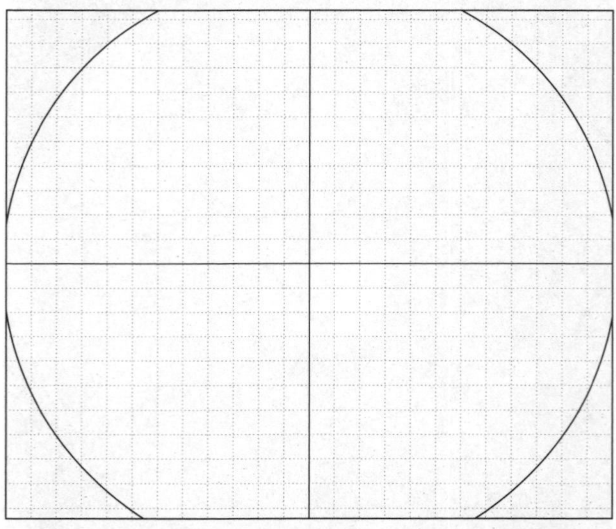

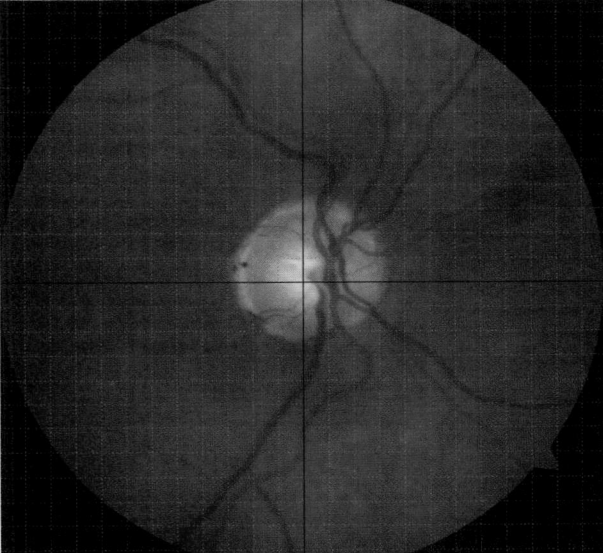

Average size nerve with subtle temporal pallor that extends beyond the cupping. Interocular and intraocular optic nerve evaluation is helpful in detecting optic nerve pallor.

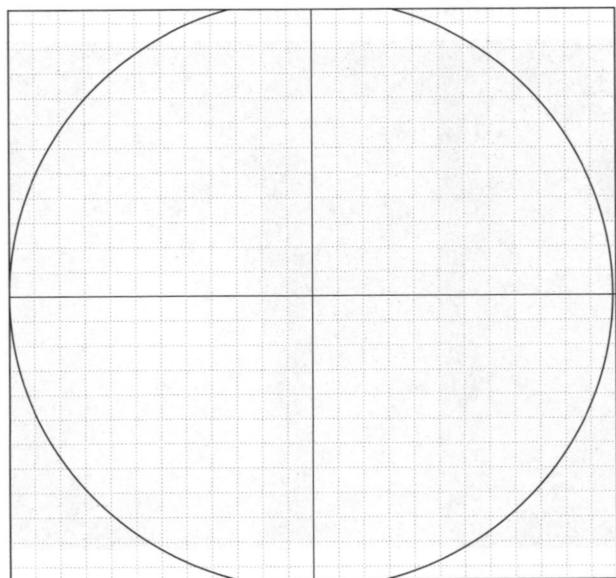

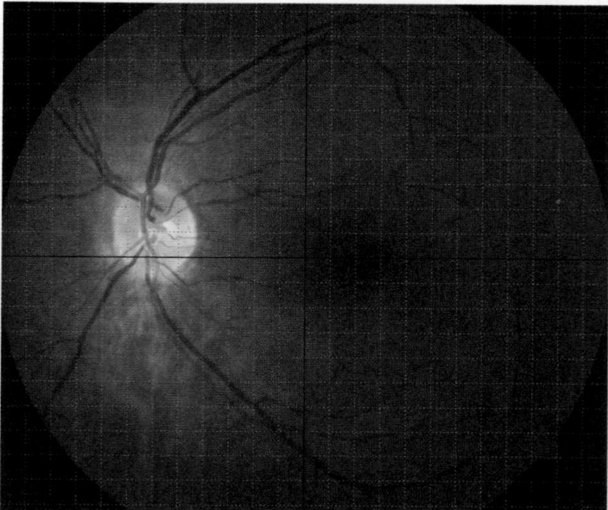

Average-small nerve with mild inferior diffuse pallor that extends beyond the small cupping. Interocular and intraocular optic nerve evaluation is helpful in detecting optic nerve pallor.

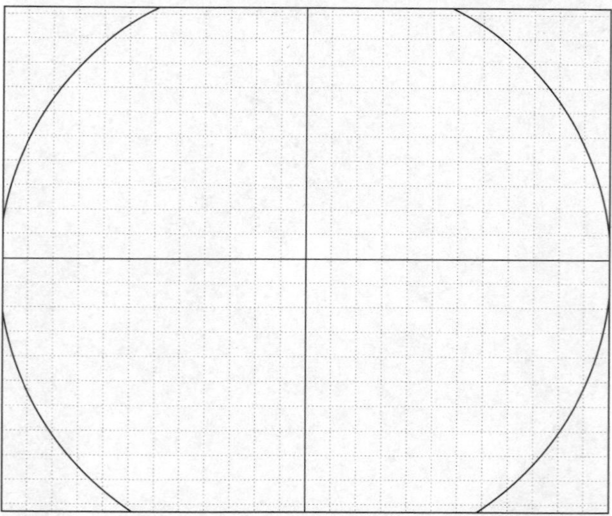

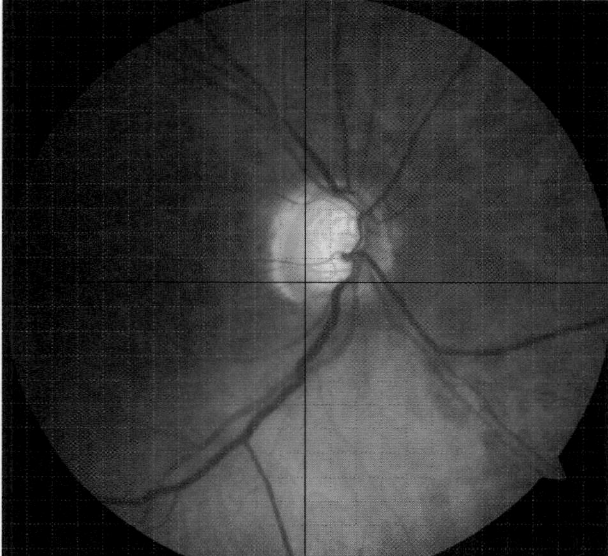

Average size nerve with superior rim thinning. Note: Normal rim perfusion despite significant cupping.

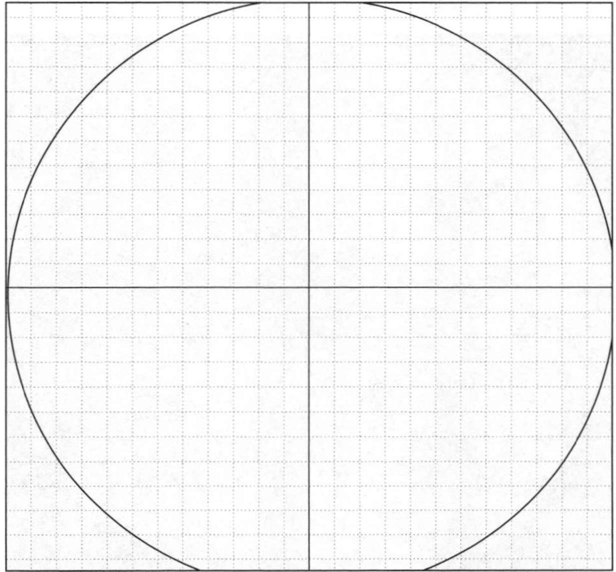

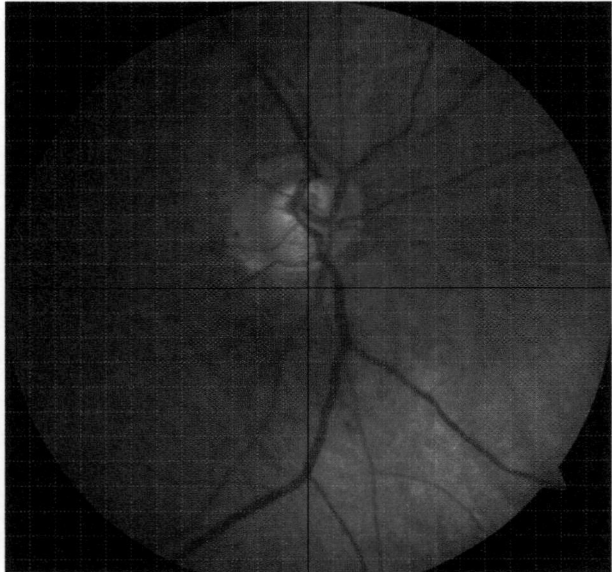

Average size nerve with inferior rim thinning. Note: Normal rim perfusion despite significant cupping.

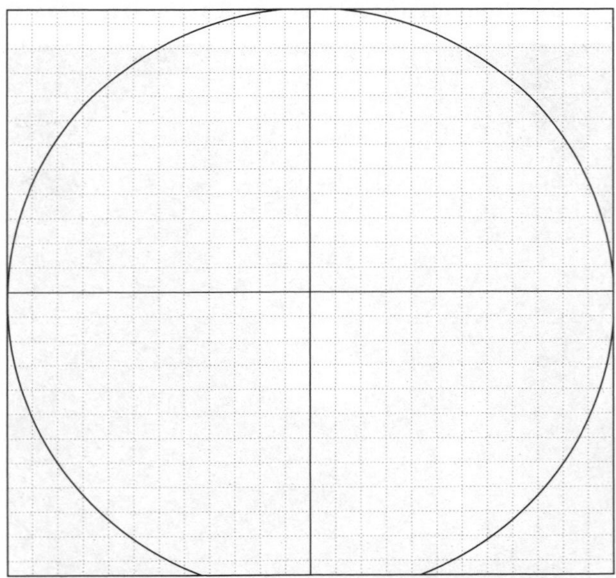

7. CENTRAL RETINAL VESSEL TRUNK LOCATION

Overview

The distance between the central retinal vessel trunk exit location and the neuroretinal rim may contribute to the vulnerability of associated glaucomatous neuroretinal rim loss.

Pearls

- **The central retinal vessel trunk may act as a stabilizing (structural and vascular) element against glaucomatous changes in the lamina cribrosa.**[1–3]
    - Limits mechanical distortion and backward bowing of the lamina cribrosa in glaucoma AND/OR may provide a supportive vascular supply to the adjacent tissue.
        - The lamina cribrosa shows more backward bowing in the inferior and superior disc sectors than close to the base of the central retinal vessel trunk.
            - Creates a "W-Shaped" lamina cribrosa appearance.
                - Example: Superior nasal vessel trunk decentration may lead to more easily deformed inferior temporal sector compared to the superior nasal sector.
        - The greater the distance between the base of the central retinal vessel trunk and the neuroretinal rim, the greater the associated glaucomatous neuroretinal rim loss, corresponding parapapillary atrophy size and enlargement, and corresponding visual field loss in glaucomatous eyes compared to normal eyes.
            - The *pattern* of glaucomatous rim loss may be associated with the distance between the central retinal vessel trunk location and the neuroretinal rim.[2–3]
            - The *pattern* of papillomacular bundle retinal nerve fiber loss is strongly correlated with, and directly proportional to, the location of the central retinal vessel trunk and the papillomacular bundle.[4]

  - The *pattern* of advanced visual field loss is correlated with the location of the central retinal vessel trunk in advanced glaucoma.[5]
  - Examine carefully those areas of the neuroretinal rim that is the greatest distance from the location of the central retinal vessel trunk and has the greatest area of parapapillary atrophy for early glaucomatous neuroretinal rim loss.[6]
- The distance between the base of the central retinal vessel trunk and the neuroretinal rim can be one of the contributing factors partially affecting local susceptibility of neuroretinal rim loss.
  - The greater the distance of the central retinal vessel trunk with respect to the neuroretinal rim, the greater the likelihood of glaucomatous neuroretinal rim loss in the associated neuroretinal rim sector.[7]

References

1. Jonas JB, Budde WM, Panda-Jonas S. Ophthalmoscopic evaluation of the optic nerve head. *Surv Ophthalmol.* 1999;43:293–320.
2. Huang H, Jonas JB, Dai Y, et al. Position of the central retinal vessel trunk and pattern of remaining visual field in advanced glaucoma. *Br J Ophthalmol.* 2013;97:96–100.
3. Jonas JB, Fernandez MC. Shape of the neuroretinal rim and position of the central retinal vessels in glaucoma.*Br J Ophthalmol.* 1994;78:99–102.
4. Rao A, Mukherjee S, Padhy D. Optic nerve head characteristics in eyes with papillomacular bundle defects in glaucoma. *Int Ophthalmol.* 2015;35(6):819–826.
5. Huang H, Jonas J, Sun X, et al. Position of the central retinal vessel trunk and pattern of remaining visual field in advanced glaucoma. *Br J Ophthalmol.* 2013;97(1):96–100.
6. Jonas J, Budde W, Németh J, et al. Central retinal vessel trunk exit and location of glaucomatous parapapillary atrophy in glaucoma. *Ophthalmology.* 2001;108:1059–1064.
7. Jonas J, Fernández M. Shape of the neuroretinal rim and position of the central retinal vessels in glaucoma. *Br J Ophthalmol.* 1994;78(2):99–102.

Further Reading

1. Wang M, Wang H, Elze T, et al. Relationship between central retinal vessel trunk location and visual field loss in glaucoma. American Journal of Ophthalmology. January 4, 2017 [Epub ahead of print].

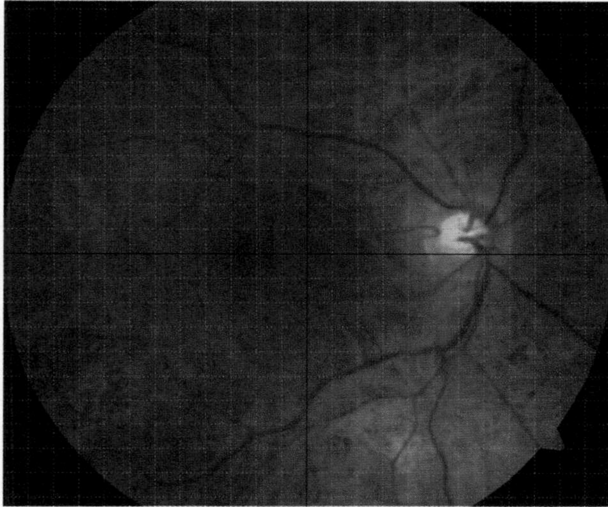

Average size nerve with moderate depth.

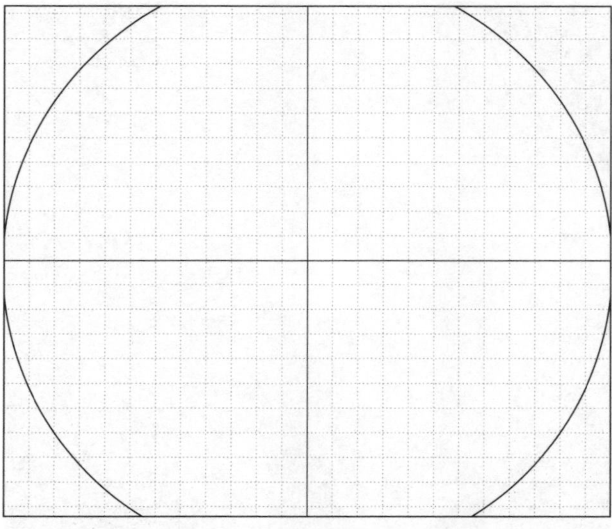

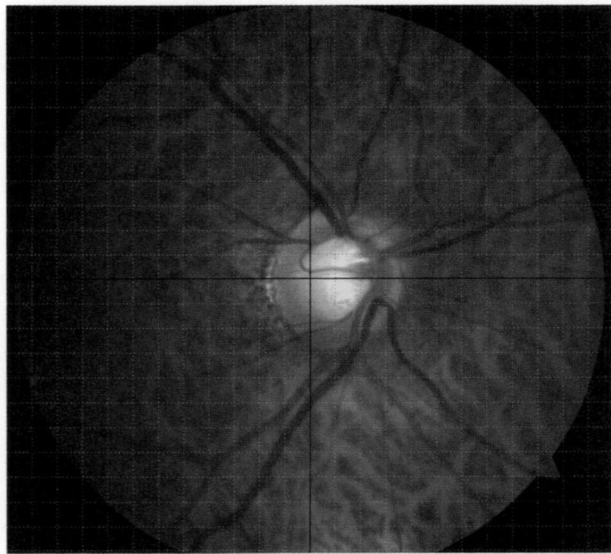

Average size nerve with central vessel trunk nasalization, vertical cupping, and moderate depth.

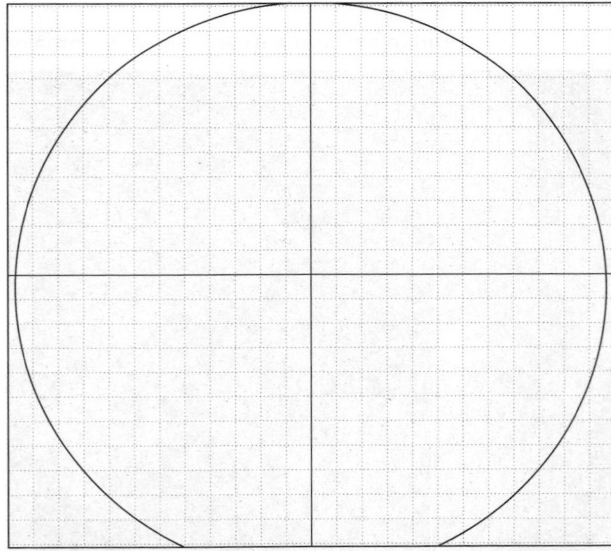

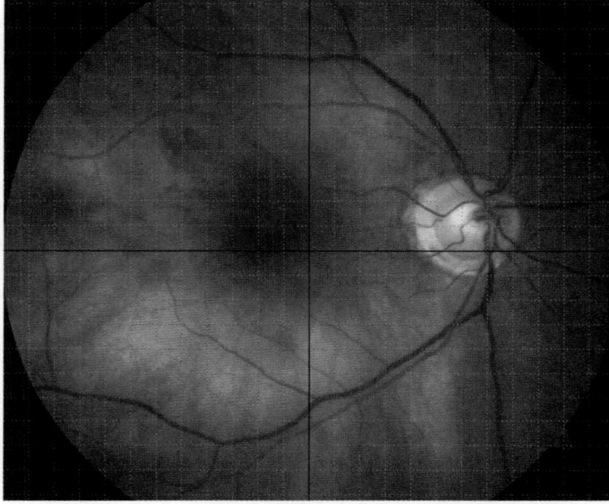

Average size nerve with superior-nasal central vessel trunk location, inferior-temporal rim thinning, and associated inferior-temporal parapapillary atrophy.

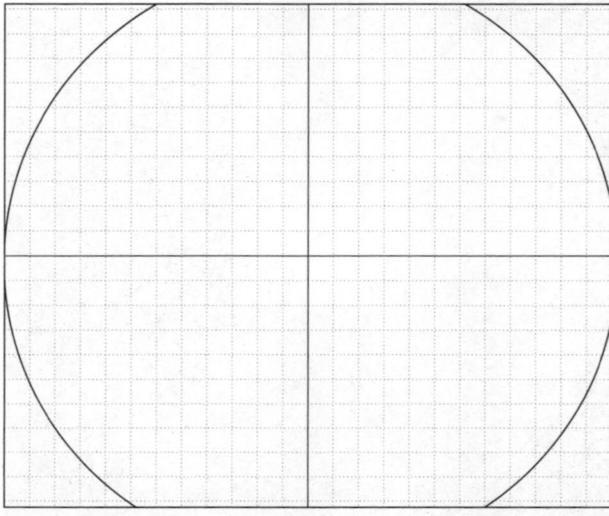

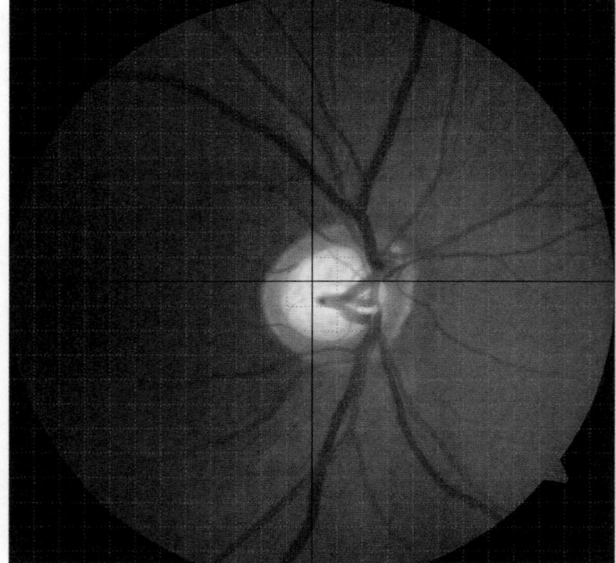

Average-large size nerve with moderate depth and large cupping.

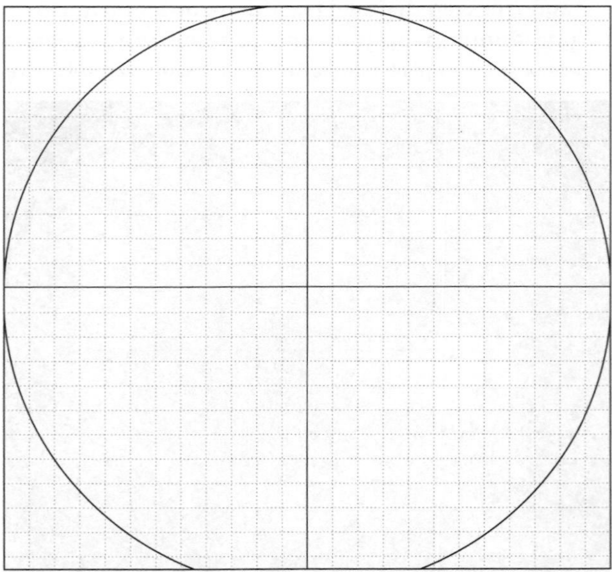

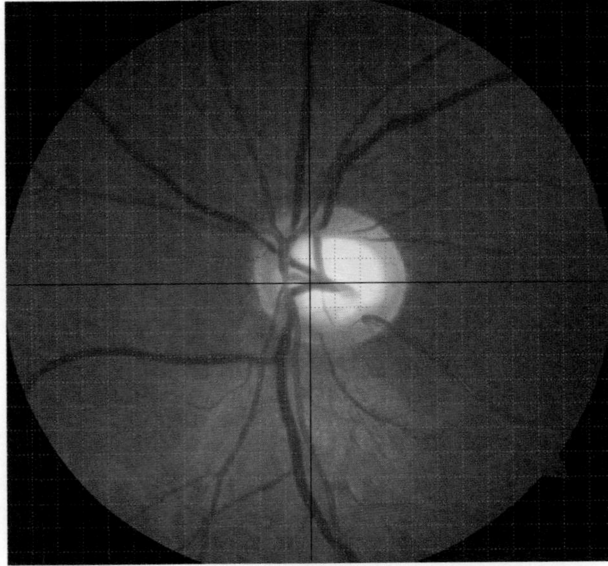

Average-large size nerve with moderate depth, large cupping, and even rim.

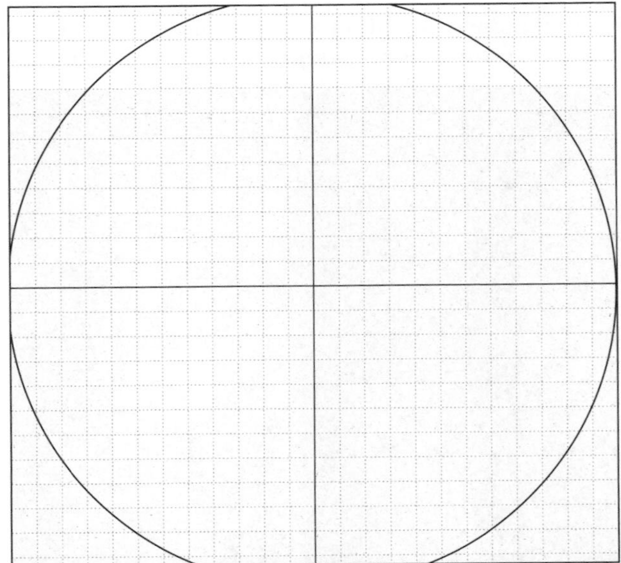

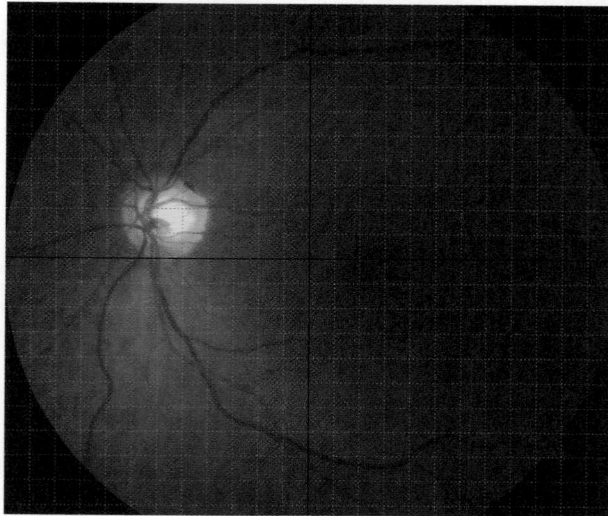

Average size nerve with inferior-nasal central vessel trunk location and associated superior-temporal rim thinning.

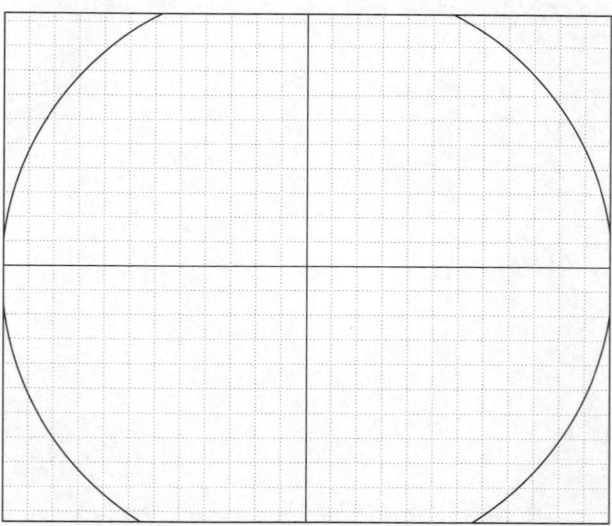

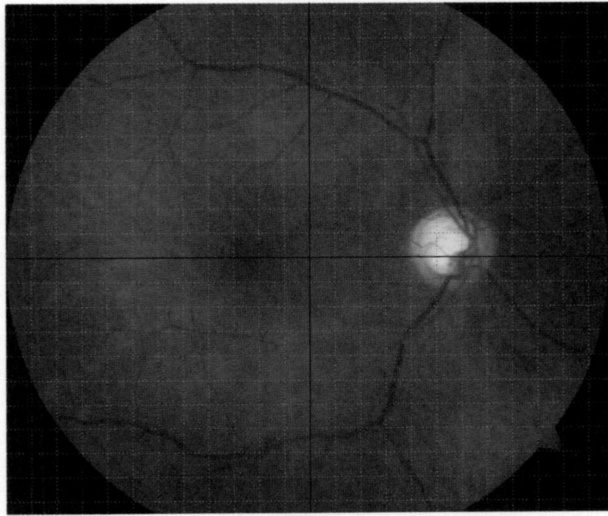

Average size nerve with inferior-nasal central vessel trunk location and associated superior-temporal rim thinning.

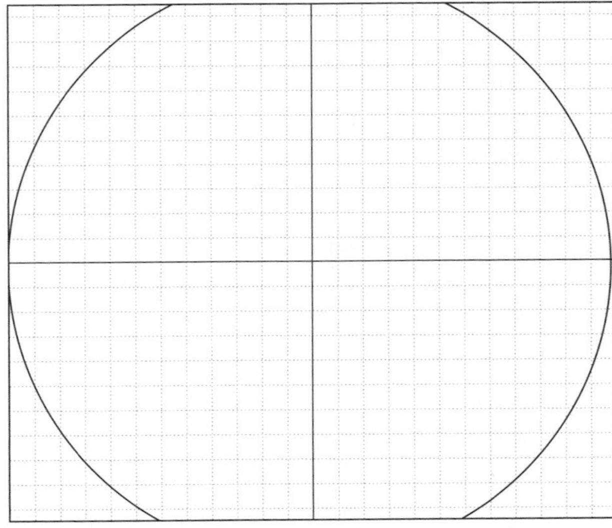

8. OPTIC DISC HEMORRHAGES

Overview

Optic disc hemorrhages have relatively high specificity but relatively low sensitivity for glaucoma.[1] These disc hemorrhages can be easily missed in routine clinical examinations,[2] have proven to be an important risk factor for the development of glaucoma in patients with ocular hypertension,[2] are a risk factor for glaucoma progression in patients who have already developed glaucoma,[3,4] and are a significant predictor for visual field loss[5] with a faster rate of visual field progression.[6] Even on a cellular level, there is evidence to suggest that eyes with glaucoma *with* disc hemorrhages have a faster rate of retinal ganglion cell loss than eyes with glaucoma that do not have disc hemorrhages.[7]

Intraocular pressure reduction can help slow glaucomatous progression following disc hemorrhages.[8]

Pearls

- **Prevalence and incidence[1]:**
  - High specificity:
    - Normal population: 0% to 1.4%
      - Disc hemorrhages are rarely found in normal eyes.
    - Other optic nerve diseases can have disc hemorrhages:
      - Posterior vitreous detachment, optic disc drusen, retinal vascular occlusive diseases, and systemic conditions (diabetes, hypertension, leukemia, systemic lupus erythematous).
  - Low sensitivity:
    - Ocular hypertension/glaucoma: 2% to 33.4%.
      - Disc hemorrhages are not found in *all* patients with ocular hypertension or glaucoma.
        - Not a reliable biomarker in screening for glaucoma.
        - Less frequent in patients with juvenile-onset primary open-angle glaucoma (POAG), age-related atrophic POAG, and highly myopic POAG.
          - ◇ Primary angle-closure prevalence: 0.5% to 5.7%.

- All prevalence estimates are more likely *a fraction of the total* of all disc hemorrhages.
  - Frequency *increases* in the early stages of glaucoma to moderate glaucoma and then *decreases* with advanced stages of glaucoma.
    - In early glaucoma, glaucomatous disc hemorrhages are usually located in the inferior temporal and superior temporal disc sectors and do not occur in advanced glaucoma in disc sectors where the neuroretinal rim is absent.[1]
- Detection can be *more frequent* by *more careful* clinical examinations and stereoscopic disc photos.

- **Appearance:**
  - Splinter-shaped/flame-shaped hemorrhages usually located at the border of, and perpendicular to, the optic disc.
    - Usually thin in appearance.
      - Flame- or fan-shaped; more likely *if* abundant vascular extravasation.
    - Can be located within the optic disc tissue (laminar or prelaminar due to laminar pore tissue remodeling and common in myopic eyes), on the neuroretinal rim, or in the parapapillary zone.
      - Usually located more in the inferior temporal and/or superior temporal areas of the optic disc.
      - Parapapillary disc hemorrhages are more likely associated with retinal nerve fiber layer (RNFL) defects and neuroretinal rim thinning.
        - Shape consistent with the orientation of the (RNFL) axons.

- **Duration:**
  - Visible for 8 days to 12 weeks after the initial bleeding.
    - Duration of glaucomatous disc hemorrhage may be associated with intraocular pressure.[1]
      - Higher intraocular pressure (IOP) may limit the extent of extravasation, resulting in smaller disc hemorrhages with potentially more rapid resolution and perhaps relatively lower perceived incidence.
      - Lower IOP may not limit the extent of extravasation, resulting in larger disc hemorrhages with potentially slower resolution and perhaps relatively higher perceived incidence.
        - Glaucomatous disc hemorrhages are most often observed in glaucoma patients with lower IOP (two to five times as much) than those with higher IOP.

- **Diagnostic importance:**
  - Glaucomatous disc hemorrhages may indicate an ongoing glaucomatous process that is present both before and after the disc hemorrhage.[9]

- IOP reduction can help slow glaucomatous progression following disc hemorrhages.[8]
- Glaucomatous disc hemorrhages are the single most significant predictor for visual field progression, and its significance and presence may be underestimated.[10,11]

References

1. Jonas JB, Budde WM, Panda-Jonas S. Ophthalmoscopic evaluation of the optic nerve head. *Surv Ophthalmol.* 1999;43:293–320.
2. Budenz D, Anderson D, Kass M, et al. Detection and prognostic significance of optic disc hemorrhages during the ocular hypertension treatment study. *Ophthalmology*. 2006;113:2137–2143.
3. Leske MC, Heijl A, Hussein M, et al. Factors for glaucoma progression and the effect of treatment: the early manifest glaucoma trial. *Arch Ophthalmol.* 2003;121(1):48–56.
4. The effectiveness of intraocular pressure reduction in the treatment of normal-tension glaucoma. Collaborative Normal-Tension Glaucoma Study Group. *Am J Ophthalmol.* 1998;126(4):498–505.
5. De Moraes CG, Liebmann JM, Park SC, et al. Optic disc progression and rates of visual field change in treated glaucoma. *Acta Ophthalmol.* 2013;91(2):e86–e91.
6. Medeiros FA, Alencar LM, Sample PA, et al. The relationship between intraocular pressure reduction and rates of progressive visual field loss in eyes with optic disc hemorrhage. *Ophthalmology.* 2010;117:2061–2066.
7. Gracitelli C, Tatham A, Zangwill L, et al. Estimated rates of retinal ganglion cell loss in glaucomatous eyes with and without optic disc hemorrhages. *PLoS ONE.* 2014;9(8):e105611.
8. Suh M, Park K. Pathogenesis and clinical implications of optic disk hemorrhage in glaucoma. *Sur Ophthalmol.* 2014;59:19–29.
9. Chung E, Demetriades A, Christos P, et al. Structural glaucomatous progression before and after occurrence of an optic disc haemorrhage. *Br J Ophthalmol.* 2015;99(1):21.
10. De Moraes C, Liebmann J, Ritch R, et al. Optic disc progression and rates of visual field change in treated glaucoma. *Acta Ophthalmol.* 2013;91(2):e86–e91.
11. De Moraes C, Liebmann J, Ritch R. Predictive factors within the optic nerve complex for glaucoma progression: disc hemorrhage and parapapillary atrophy. *Asia-Pacific J Ophthalmol.* 2012;1(2):105–112.

Further Reading

1. Drance S, Fairclough M, Butler D, et al. The importance of disc hemorrhage in the prognosis of chronic open angle glaucoma. *Arch Ophthalmol.* 1977;95(2):226–228.
2. Sonnsjö B, Dokmo Y, Krakau T. Disc haemorrhages, precursors of open angle glaucoma. *Prog Retin Eye Res.* 2002;21:35–56.
3. Uhler T, Piltz-Seymour J. Optic disc hemorrhages in glaucoma and ocular hypertension: implications and recommendations. *Curr Opin Ophthalmol.* 2008;19(2):89–94.
4. Healey P, Mitchell P, Smith W, et al. Optic disc hemorrhages in a population with and without signs of glaucoma. *Ophthalmology.* 1998;105(2):216–223.

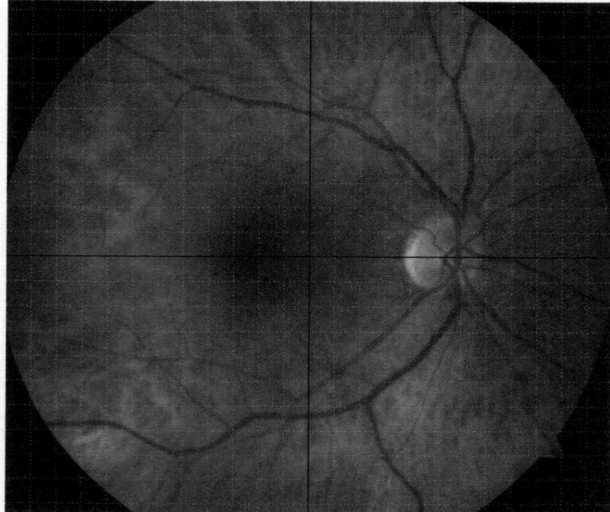

Small nerve with inferior, nonglaucomatous disc hemorrhage.

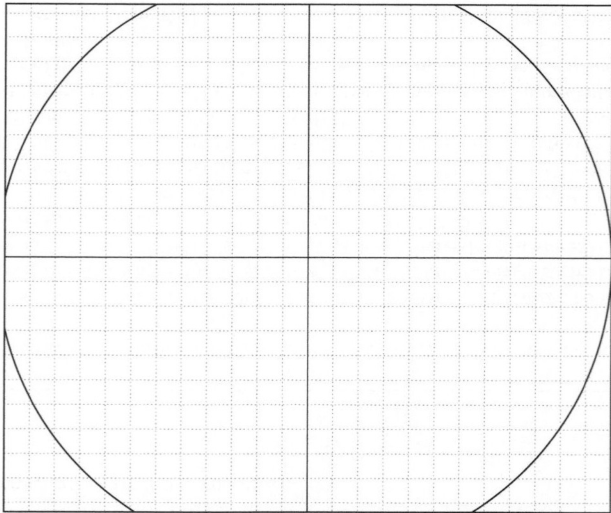

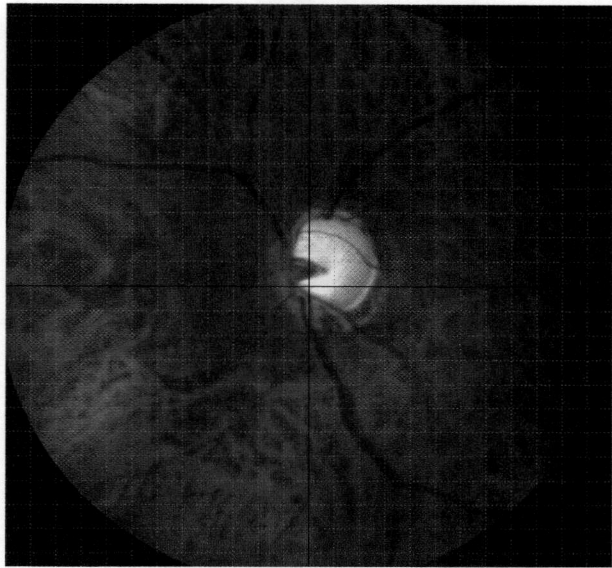

End-stage glaucoma with inferior glaucomatous disc hemorrhage adjacent to remaining rim tissue.

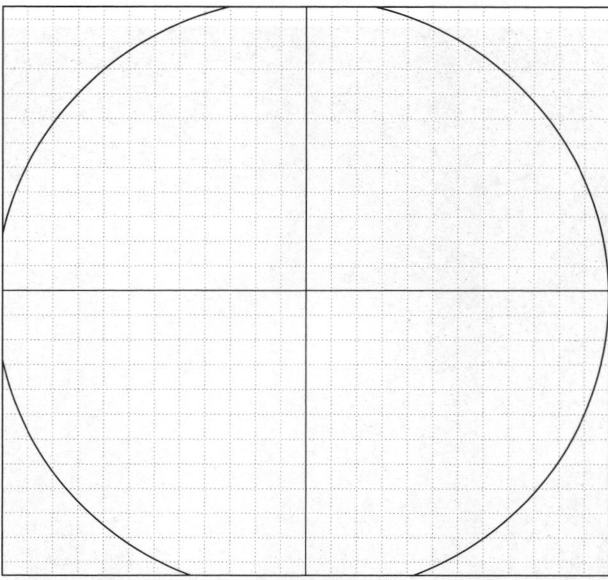

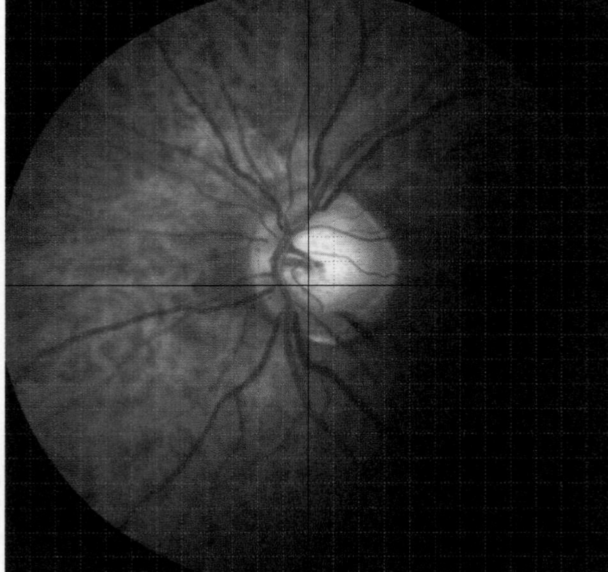

Average-large size nerve with inferior temporal glaucomatous disc hemorrhage, associated rim thinning, retinal arteriole narrowing, and parapapillary atrophy.

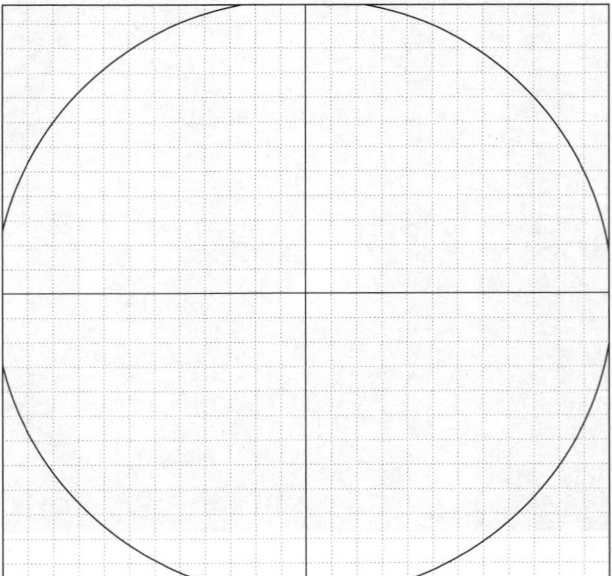

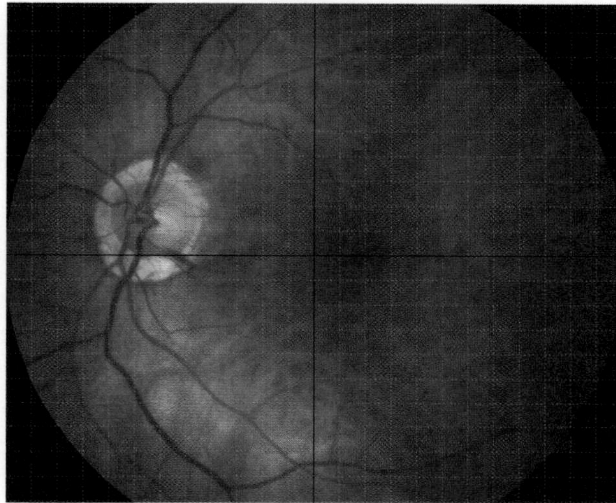

Average size nerve with inferior temporal glaucomatous disc hemorrhage, associated rim thinning, and parapapillary atrophy.

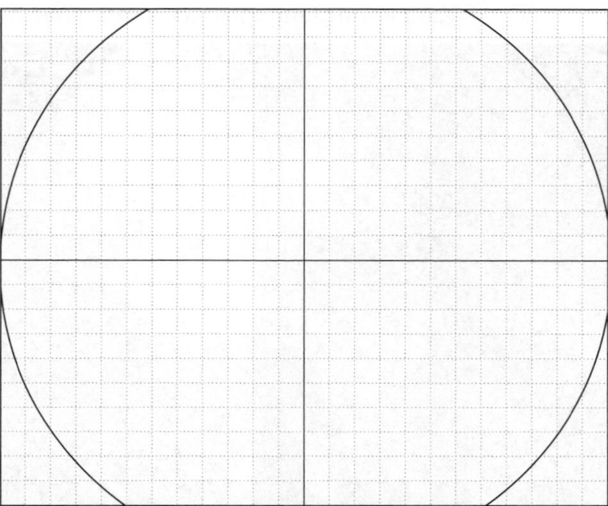

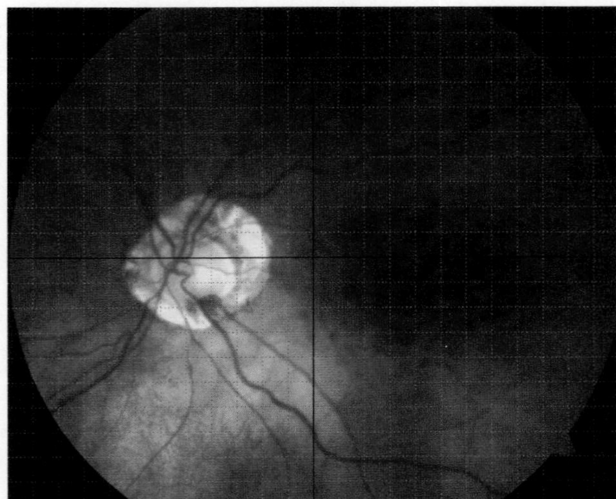

Average size nerve with inferior temporal glaucomatous disc hemorrhage, associated rim thinning, and diffuse parapapillary atrophy. Note: Systematic evaluation of the whole nerve for disc hemorrhages shows a subtle glaucomatous disc hemorrhage located superior-temporally. If you see one disc hemorrhage, be sure to look for others too.

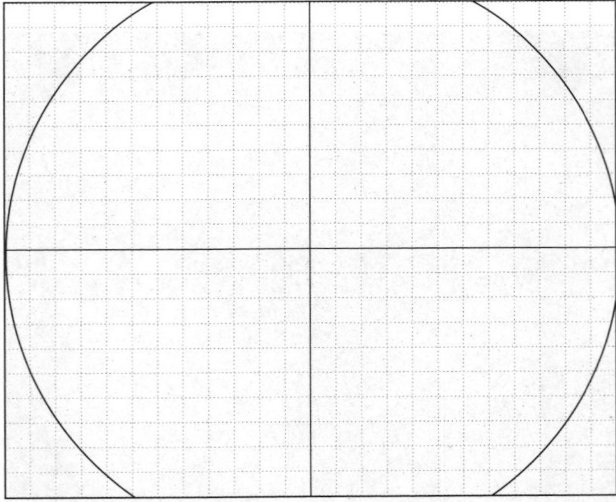

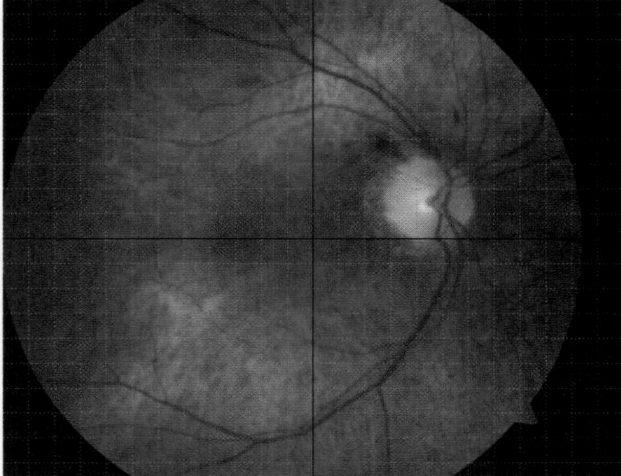

Average size nerve with moderate temporal pallor, nonglaucomatous disc hemorrhage, and retinal hemorrhages.

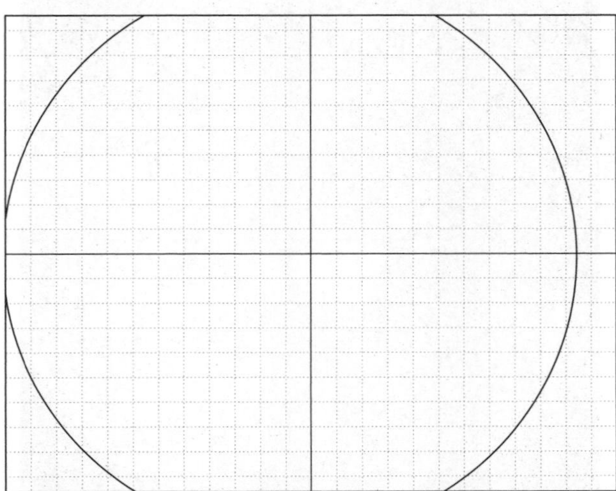

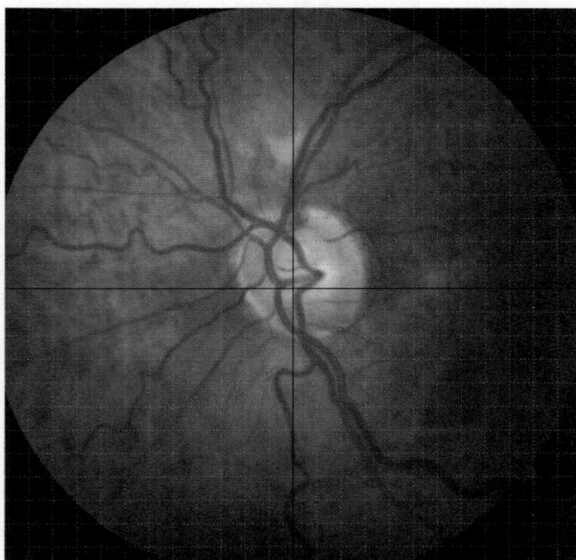

Average-large size nerve with subtle glaucomatous disc hemorrhages on the inferior and superior neuroretinal rim with associated thinning and retinal arteriole narrowing. Note: Systematic evaluation of the whole nerve for disc hemorrhages shows a subtle glaucomatous disc hemorrhage located inferior-temporally. If you see one disc hemorrhage, be sure to look for others too.

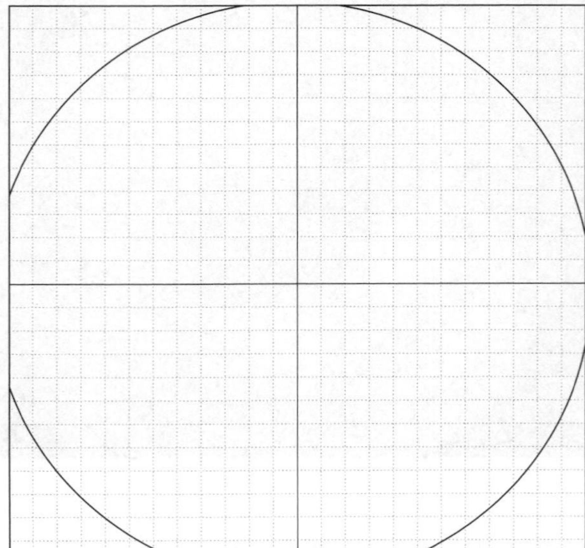

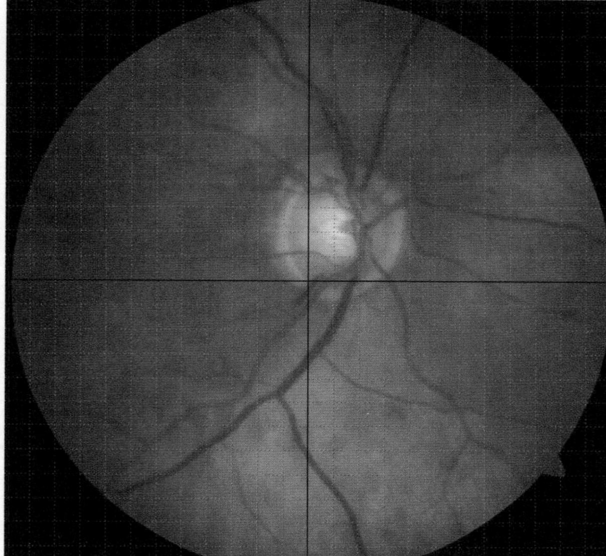

Average-large size nerve with glaucomatous disc hemorrhages on the inferior and superior neuroretinal rim with associated thinning. Note: Systematic evaluation of the whole nerve for disc hemorrhages shows a subtle glaucomatous disc hemorrhage located superior-temporally. If you see one disc hemorrhage, be sure to look for others too.

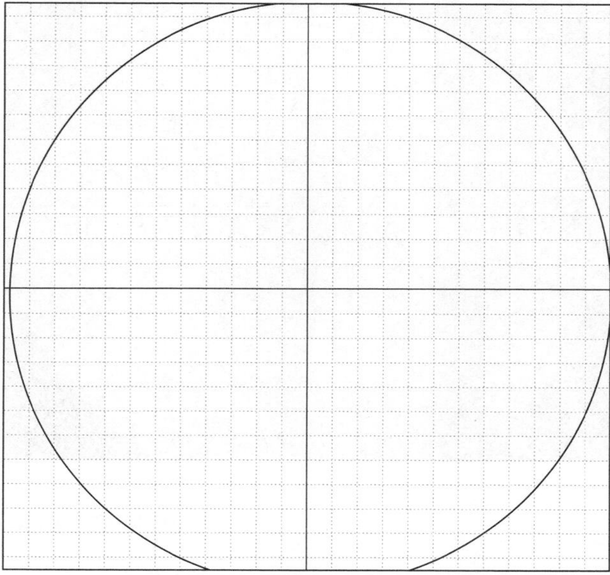

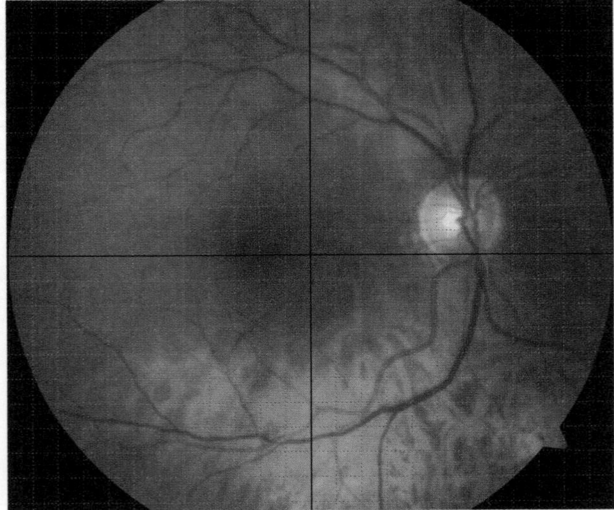

Average size nerve with subtle inferior glaucomatous disc hemorrhage.

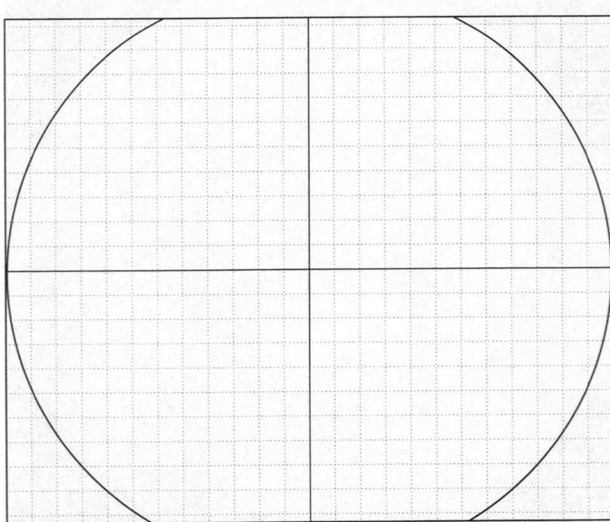

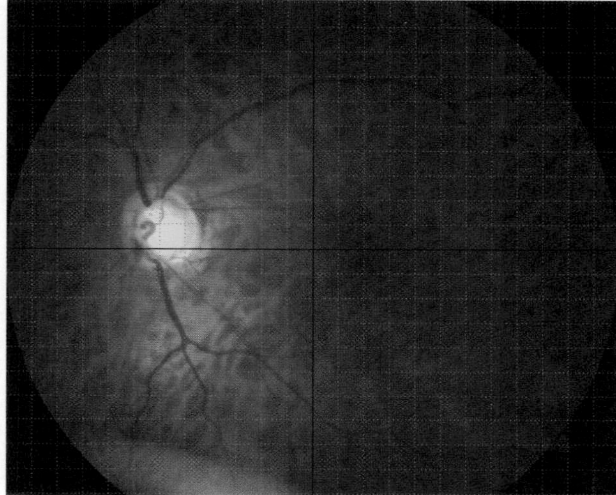

Average size nerve with glaucomatous disc hemorrhage on the remaining nasal rim. If present, and as shown in the image here, such disc hemorrhages in this location are more commonly observed in advanced glaucoma stages.

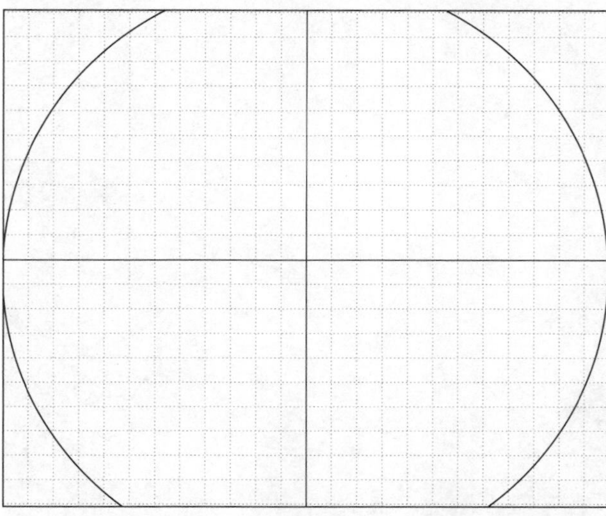

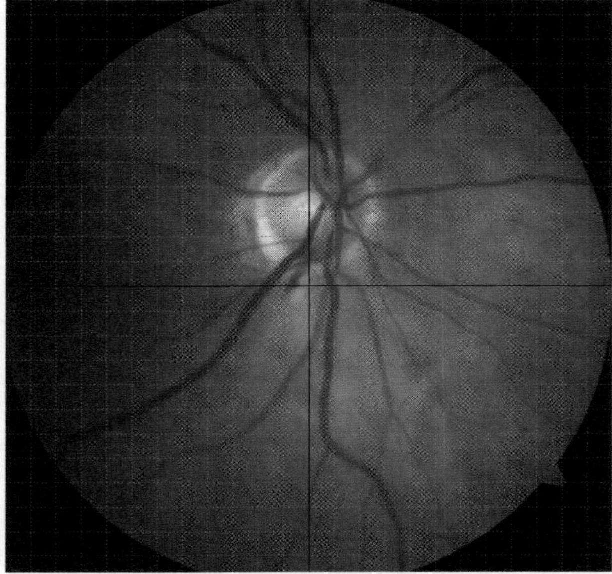

Average size nerve and glaucomatous disc hemorrhage with classic appearance and location.

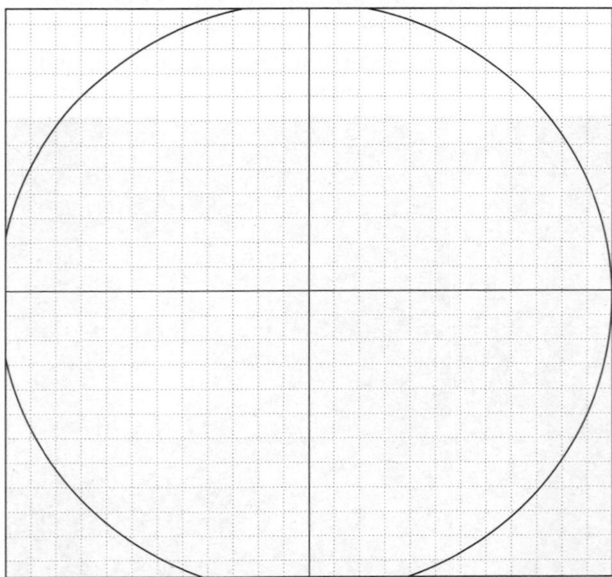

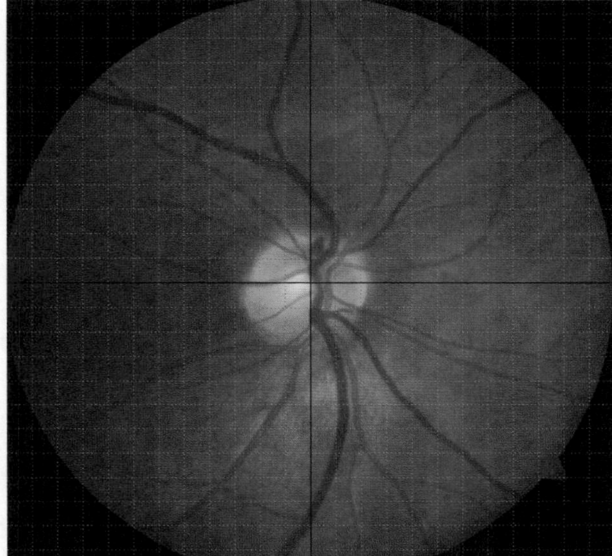

Average size nerve with likely nonglaucomatous disc hemorrhage based on overall healthy rim appearance and preserved superior retinal nerve fiber layer pattern.

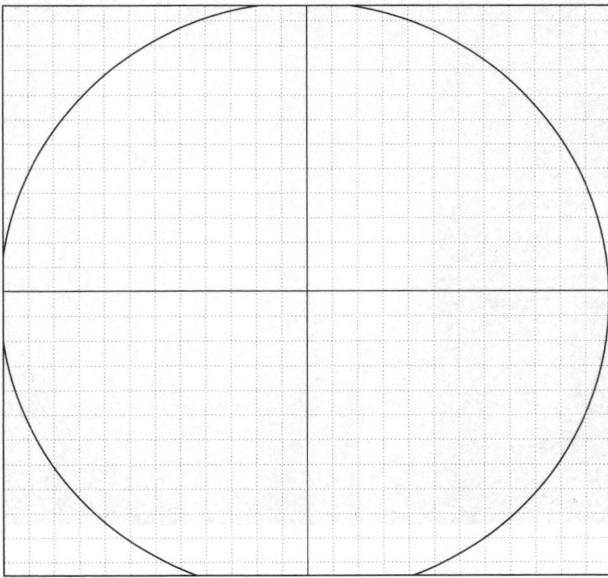

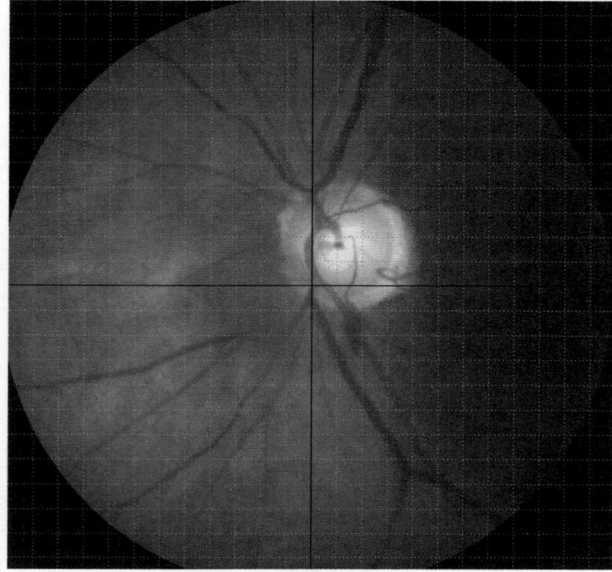

Average size nerve with inferior glaucomatous disc hemorrhage, parapapillary atrophy, and associated neuroretinal thinning.

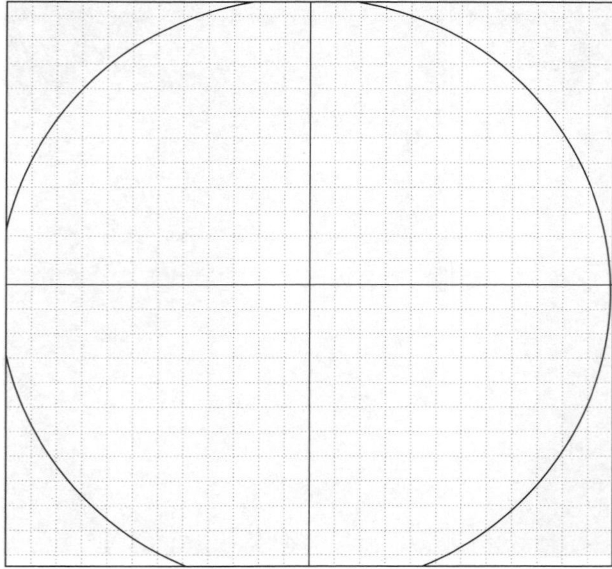

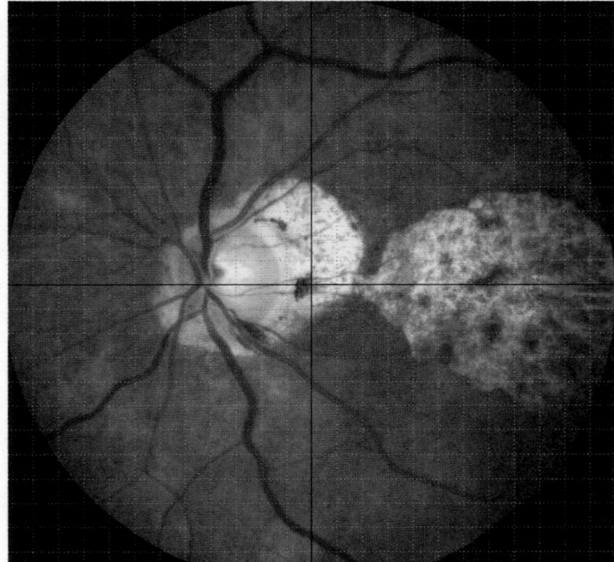

Average size nerve with inferior glaucomatous disc hemorrhage, parapapillary atrophy, and associated neuroretinal thinning as well as diffuse macular geographic atrophy.

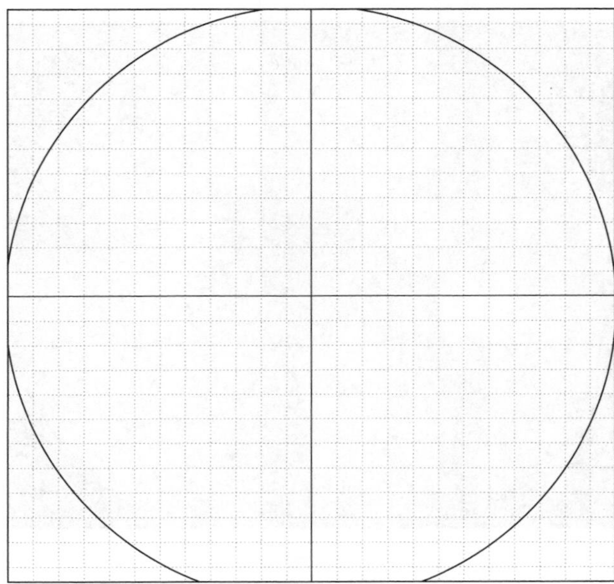

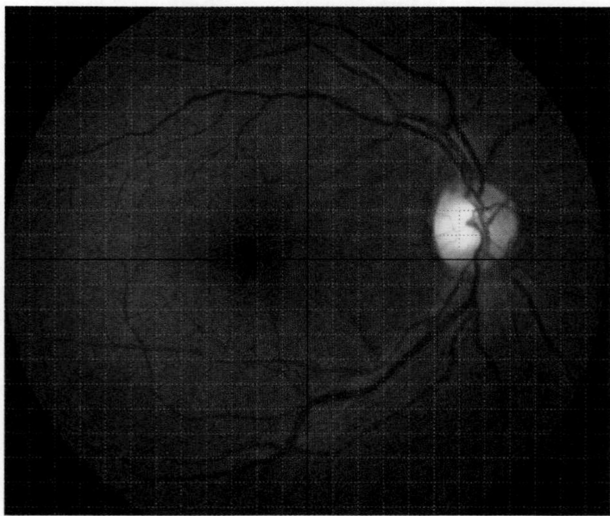

Average size nerve with subtle superior glaucomatous disc hemorrhage on the neuroretinal rim. Note: The associated superior retinal nerve fiber layer (RNFL) pattern loss relative to the more robust inferior (RNFL) pattern appearance.

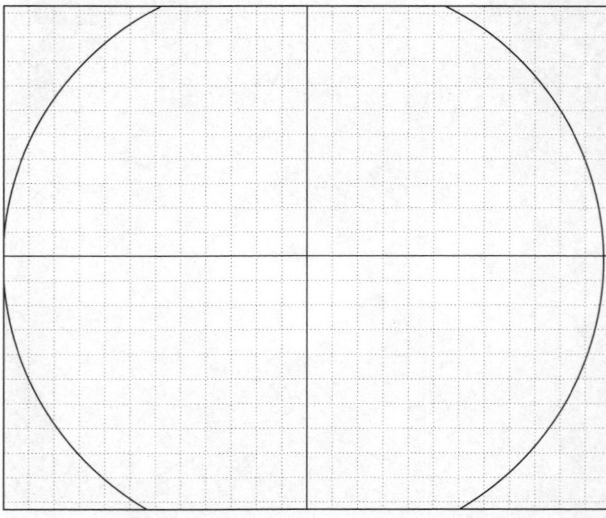

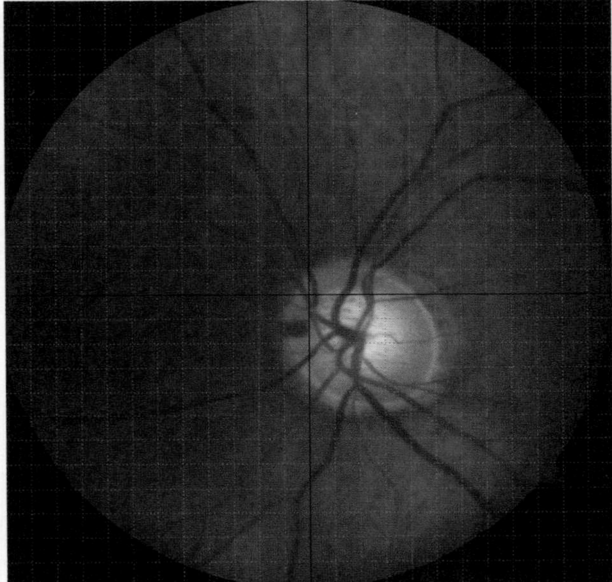

Average-large nerve with nasal glaucomatous disc hemorrhage. If present, and as shown in the image here, such disc hemorrhages in this location are more commonly observed in advanced glaucoma stages.

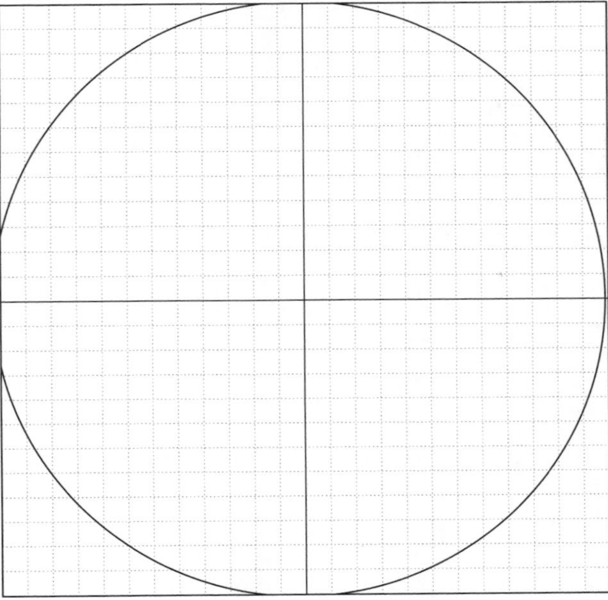

9. PARAPAPILLARY CHORIORETINAL ATROPHY

Overview

Parapapillary atrophy (PPA)[1] is more frequently observed in patients with glaucoma than in those with ocular hypertension and normal individuals.[2,3] The incidence of PPA has been found to be significantly higher in eyes with glaucomatous structural and/or functional progression compared to eyes without glaucomatous structural and/or functional progression.[2,3] PPA progression is associated with progressive structural and functional glaucomatous damage.[2,3]

The alpha and beta zones of PPA are larger in eyes with glaucoma than in eyes without glaucoma.[4–6] The frequency of beta-zone PPA is strongly correlated with the stage of the disease as well as the associated structural glaucomatous damage such as neuroretinal rim loss, decreased retinal vessel diameter, decreased retinal nerve fiber layer (RNFL) visibility, and correlating visual field defects.[4–6]

The presence of beta-zone PPA can be very helpful in the diagnosis of early glaucoma and can be a predictive factor for glaucomatous progression in those already diagnosed with glaucoma.[7,8]

PPA is important in the morphologic diagnosis of glaucomatous optic neuropathy.

Pearls

- **Appearance:**
  - In normal eyes, both alpha and beta zones are largest and most frequently located in the temporal horizontal sector followed by the inferior temporal and superior temporal sectors. This PPA is smallest and least frequently observed in the nasal parapapillary area.
  - Alpha zone:
    - Peripheral zone of irregular hypopigmentation/hyperpigmentation with chorioretinal thinning.
      - Outer border is adjacent to the retina.
      - Inner border is adjacent either to the peripapillary scleral ring or to the beta zone (visible sclera and visible large choroidal vessels).

    - Equivalent to pigmentary irregularities in the retinal pigment epithelium.
    - Found in almost ALL normal eyes (15% to 20%), therefore more common than beta zone.
    - Relative scotoma.
- Beta zone:
    - If present, beta-zone PPA is adjacent to the peripapillary scleral ring.
        - The <u>b</u>eta zone <u>b</u>orders the optic nerve.
        - Characterized by smooth margins with the adjacent alpha zone on its outer border and with the peripapillary scleral ring on its inner border.
            - If both zones are present, the beta zone is always closer to the optic disc than the alpha zone.
    - Significant RPE atrophy with easily visible sclera and large choroidal vessels.
        - Associated with significant thinning of the chorioretinal tissue and reduced choroidal volume.
            - May suggest reduced vascular perfusion in patients with primary open-angle glaucoma (POAG).[9]
            - Absolute scotoma.
    - Occurs more commonly in eyes with glaucomatous optic neuropathy than in normal eyes.
        - Size and frequency of beta-zone PPA are significantly associated with glaucomatous optic nerve head damage, neuroretinal rim loss, greatest distance from the base of the central vessel trunk, decreased retinal vessel diameter, reduced RNFL visibility, and associated visual field defects.[1,4–6]
            - The more neuroretinal rim loss, the greater the area of PPA.
            - Disc hemorrhages may be closely associated with the *size* of the PPA.
            - The presence of beta-zone PPA increases the risk of glaucoma progression AND those patients with beta-zone PPA may have a faster rate of glaucoma progression.[10]
        - Can be considered an early sign of glaucoma in patients with ocular hypertension.
            - Presence and size of PPA are related to the development of subsequent optic disc or visual field damage in patients with ocular hypertension.
    - Size:
        - Beta-zone (largest) high myopic POAG > age-related atrophic POAG > secondary open angle glaucoma (pseudoexfoliation glaucoma, pigmentary dispersion glaucoma, and low myopia POAG) > juvenile-onset POAG (smallest).
            - PPA may be larger in size in patients with normal-tension glaucoma than in patients with high-tension glaucoma.
                - "In glaucomatous eyes with high IOP, deep and steep cupping, and relatively fast development of optic nerve damage, neuroretinal rim loss may occur earlier than parapapillary atrophy can develop. . ."[1]

- The depth of the cup is slightly associated with the degree of PPA, i.e., the deeper and steeper the cup, the smaller the PPA.

- **Significance:**
  - Nonglaucomatous optic nerve damage does not lead to an enlargement of PPA.
    - One of few variables to distinguish between glaucomatous and nonglaucomatous optic nerve damage.[11]
    - The presence of beta-zone PPA is a risk factor for glaucoma progression, and its presence and significance may be underestimated.[12]
      - In Caucasians, the presence of a large area of beta-zone PPA and small neuroretinal rim size are predictive factors for glaucomatous optic nerve progression.[13]
  - Size, shape, and frequency of alpha and beta zones do not differ significantly between normal eyes and eyes with non-glaucomatous optic nerve atrophy.
    - Both zones, however, are significantly larger, and beta zones occur more often in eyes with glaucomatous optic nerve atrophy than in normal eyes.
      - Frequently gets worse (enlarges) with glaucoma progression, nonglaucomatous optic nerve damage *does not* lead to enlargement of the PPA.

References

1. Jonas JB, Budde WM, Panda-Jonas S. Ophthalmoscopic evaluation of the optic nerve head. *Surv Ophthalmol.* 1999;43:293–320.
2. Uchida H, Ugurlu S, Caprioli J. Increasing peripapillary atrophy is associated with progressive glaucoma. *Ophthalmology.* 1998;105(8):1541–1545.
3. Budde W, Jonas J. Enlargement of parapapillary atrophy in follow-up of chronic open-angle glaucoma. *Am J Ophthalmol.* 2004;137:646–654.
4. Jonas JB, Nguyen XN, Gusek GC, et al. Parapapillary chorioretinal atrophy in normal and glaucoma eyes. I. Morphometric data. *Invest Ophthalmol Vis Sci.* 1989;30:908–918.
5. Jonas JB, Naumann GO. Parapapillary chorioretinal atrophy in normal and glaucoma eyes. II. Correlations. *Invest Ophthalmol Vis Sci.* 1989;30:919–926.
6. Jonas JB. Clinical implications of peripapillary atrophy in glaucoma. *Curr Opin Ophthalmol.* 2005;16:84–88.
7. Jonas JB, Budde WM. Diagnosis and pathogenesis of glaucomatous optic neuropathy: morphological aspects. *Prog Retin Eye Res.* 2000;19:1–40.
8. Jonas J, Martus P, Horn F, et al. Predictive factors of the optic nerve head for development or progression of glaucomatous visual field loss. *Invest Ophthalmol Vis Sci.* 2004;45(8):2613–2618.
9. Sullivan-Mee M, Patel NB, Pensyl D, et al. Relationship between juxtapapillary choroidal volume and beta-zone parapapillary atrophy in eyes with and without primary open-angle glaucoma. *Am J Ophthalmol.* 2015;160(4):637–647.e1.
10. Teng C, De Moraes C, Prata T, et al. Original article: β-Zone parapapillary atrophy and the velocity of glaucoma progression. *Ophthalmology.* 2010;117:909–915.
11. Jonas J. Clinical implications of peripapillary atrophy in glaucoma. *Curr Opin Ophthalmol.* 2005;16(2):84–88.
12. De Moraes C, Liebmann J, Ritch R. Predictive factors within the optic nerve complex for glaucoma progression: disc hemorrhage and parapapillary atrophy. *Asia-Pacific J Ophthalmol.* 2012;1(2):105–112.
13. Jonas J, Martus P, Budde W, et al. Small neuroretinal rim and large parapapillary atrophy as predictive factors for progression of glaucomatous optic neuropathy. *Ophthalmology.* 2002;109:1561–1567.

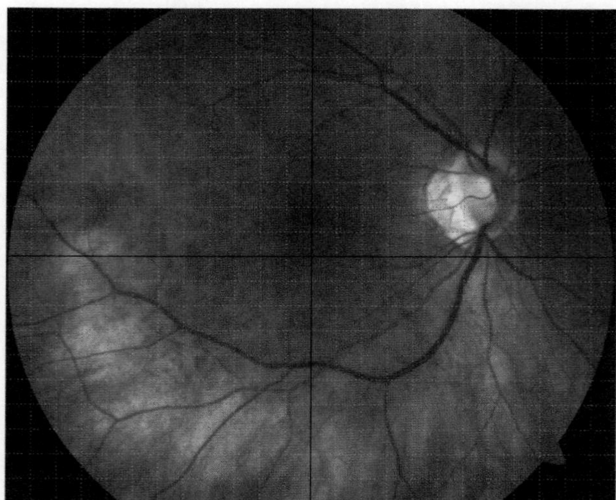

Oval-shaped nerve with tilted insertion, temporal sloping, and temporal parapapillary atrophy.

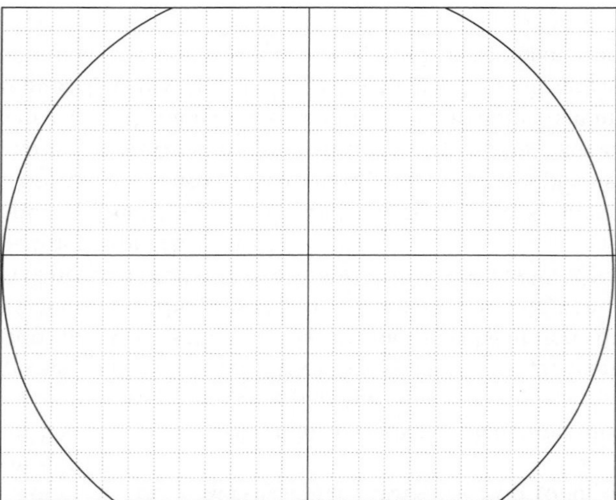

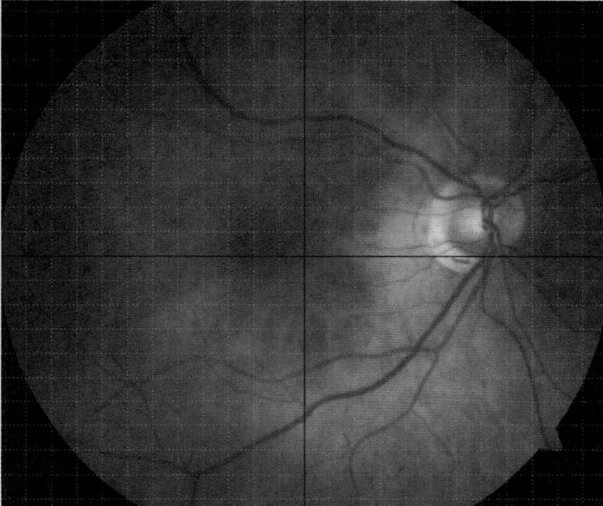

Average size nerve with temporal parapapillary atrophy.

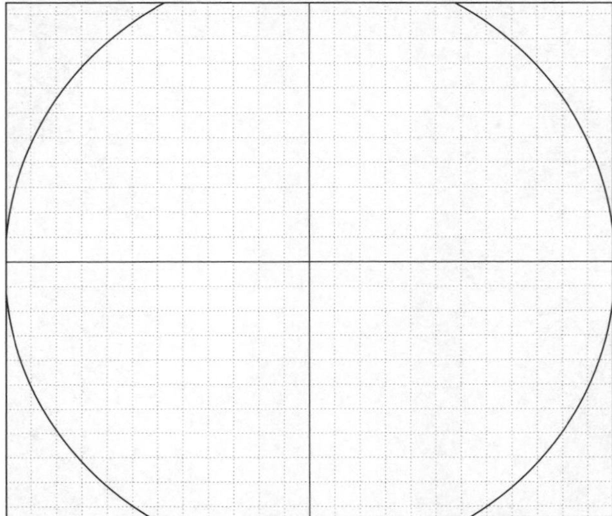

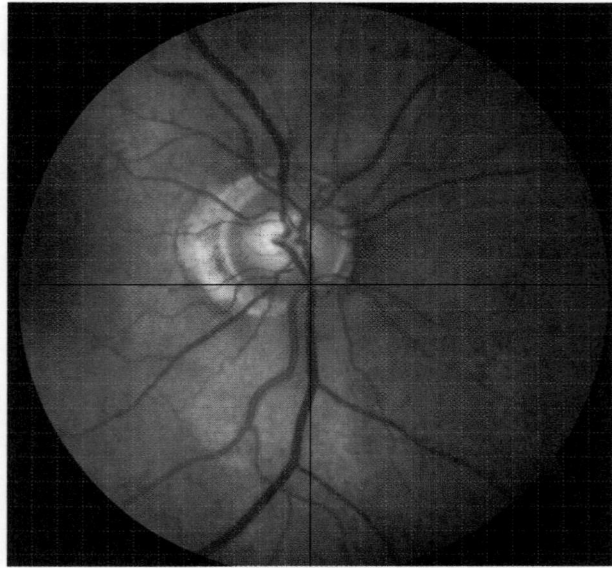

Average size nerve with peripheral alpha-zone and inner beta-zone parapapillary atrophy.

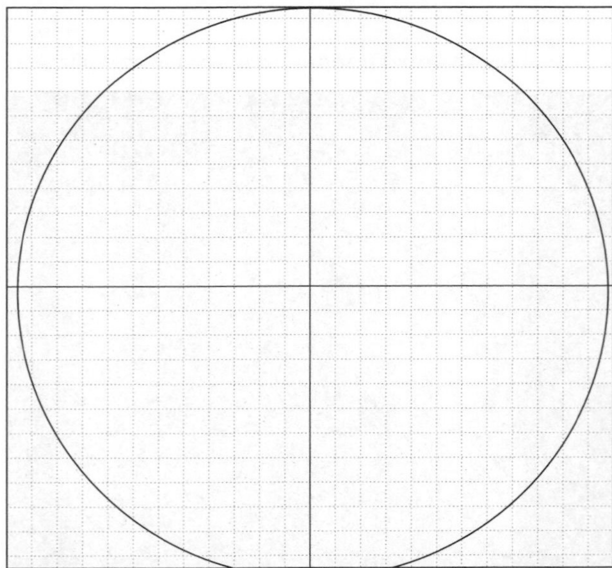

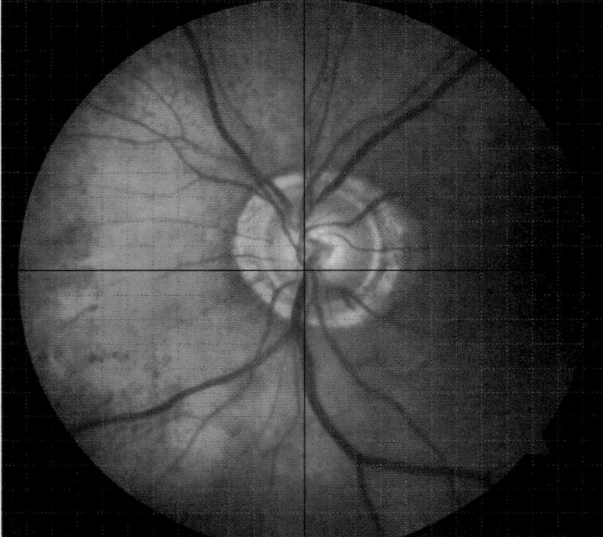

Average size nerve with temporal alpha-zone and circumferential inner beta/gamma-zone parapapillary atrophy, inferior glaucomatous disc hemorrhage, and associated inferior temporal neuroretinal rim thinning.

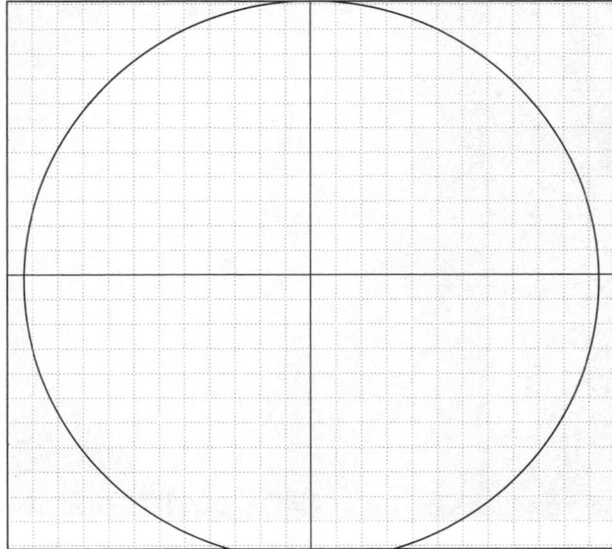

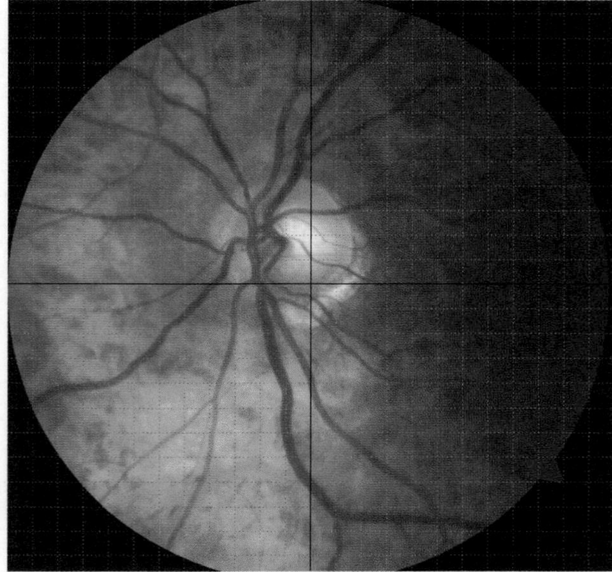

Average size nerve with inferior temporal parapapillary atrophy, associated neuroretinal rim thinning, and arteriole vessel narrowing.

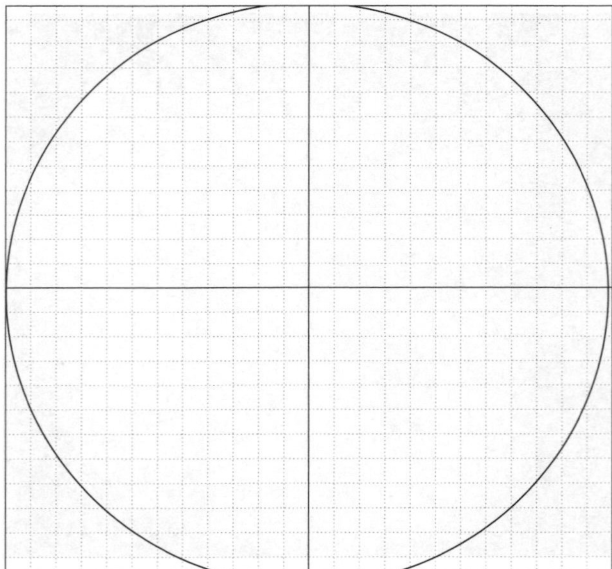

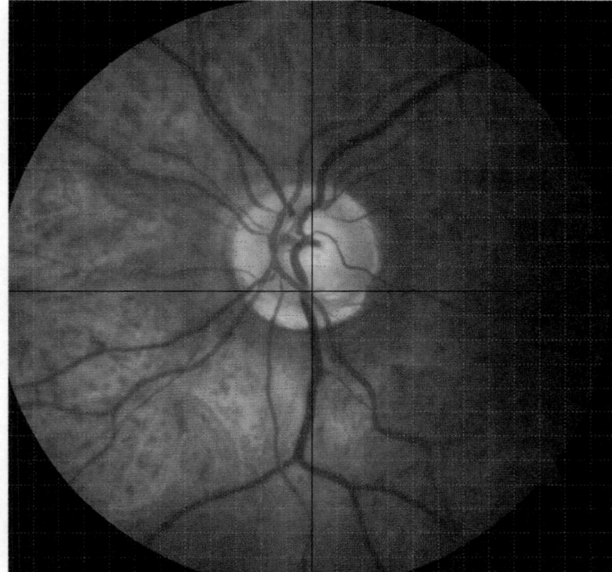

Average size nerve with inferior parapapillary atrophy and associated inferior neuroretinal rim thinning.

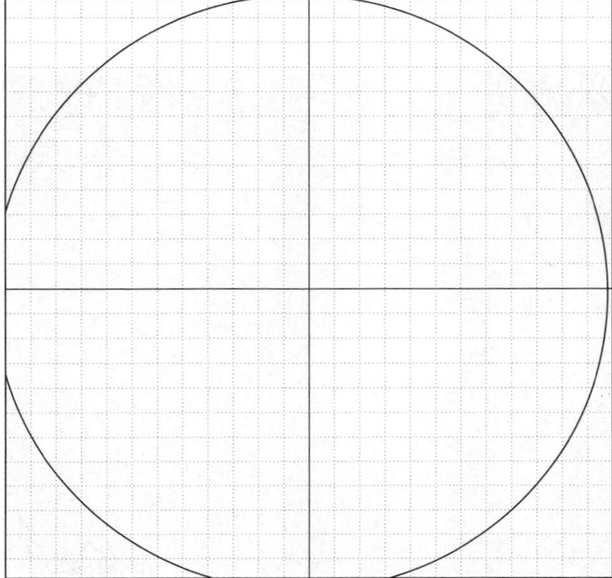

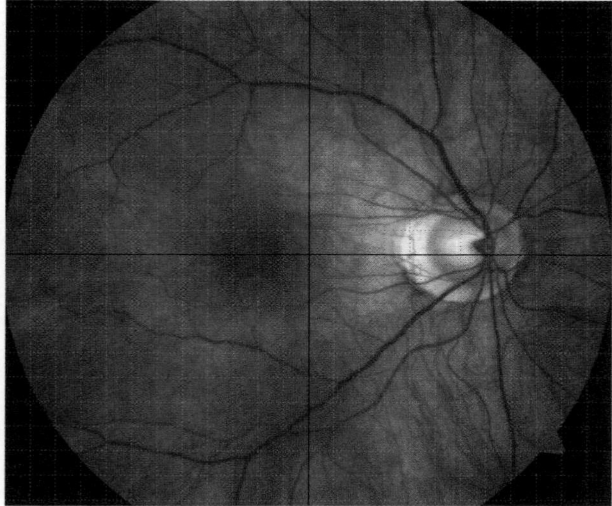

Average size nerve with inferior and temporal parapapillary atrophy.

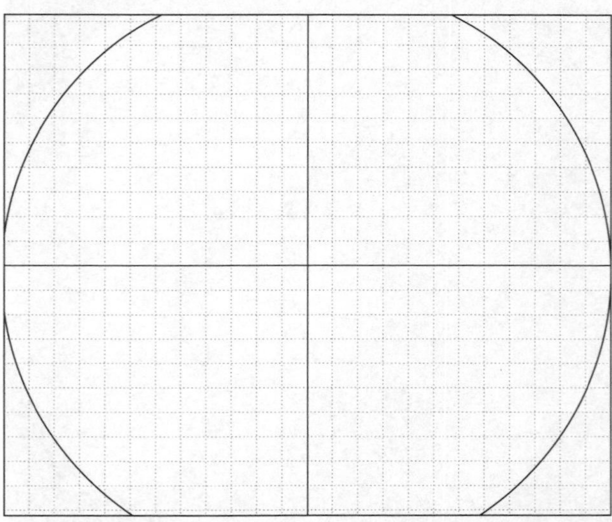

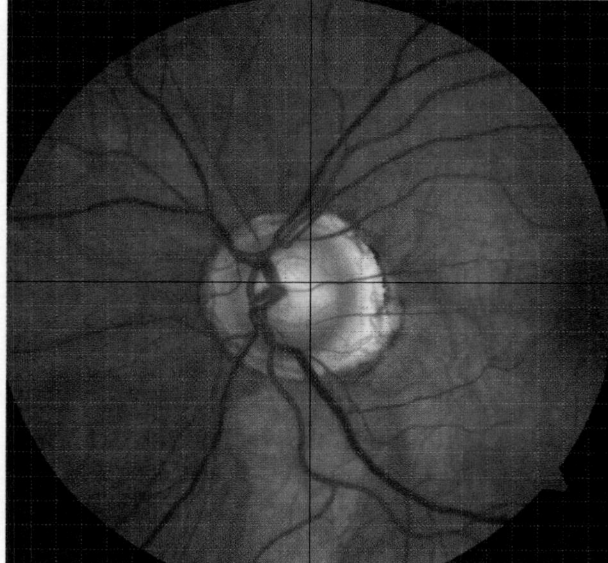

Average size nerve with parapapillary atrophy (greatest inferior-temporal), associated neuroretinal rim thinning, and arteriole vessel narrowing.

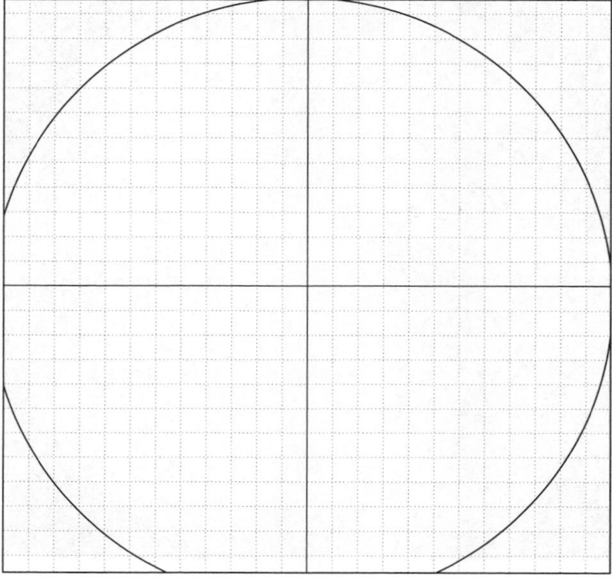

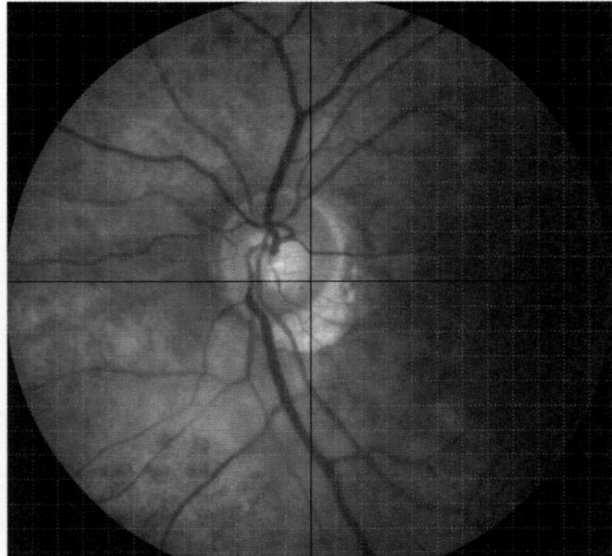

Average size nerve with parapapillary atrophy (greatest inferior-temporal), associated neuroretinal rim thinning, and arteriole vessel narrowing.

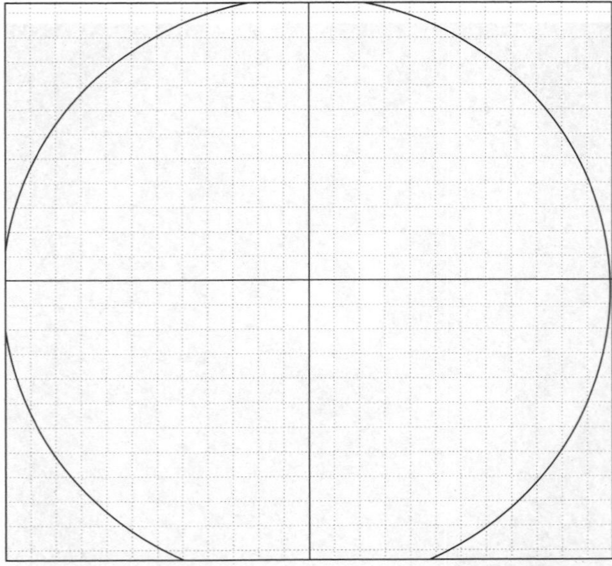

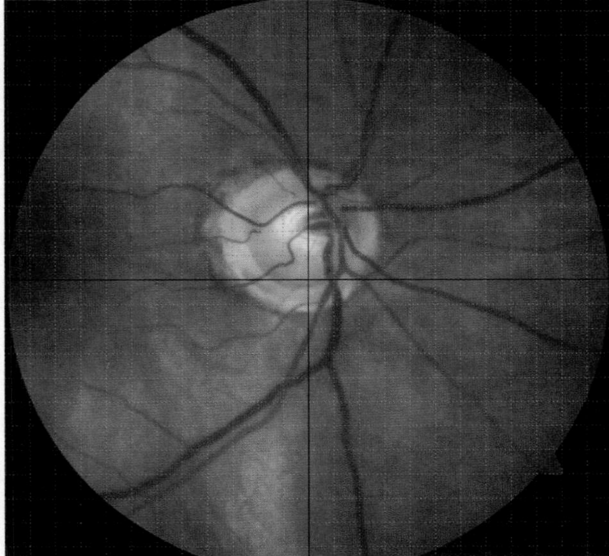

Average size nerve with peripheral alpha-zone and inner beta-zone parapapillary atrophy.

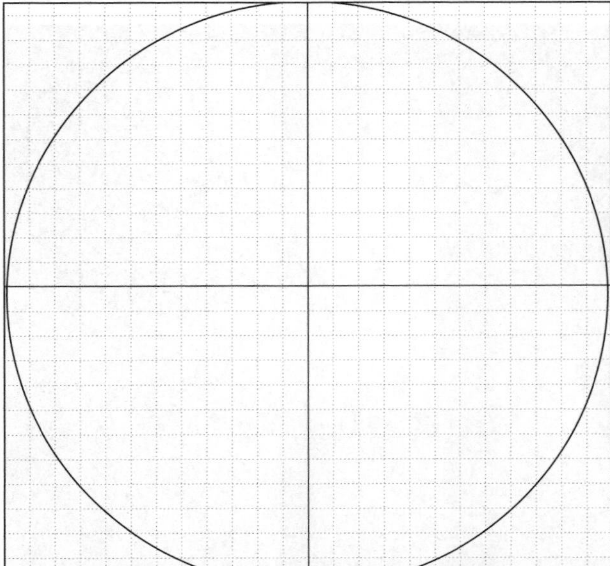

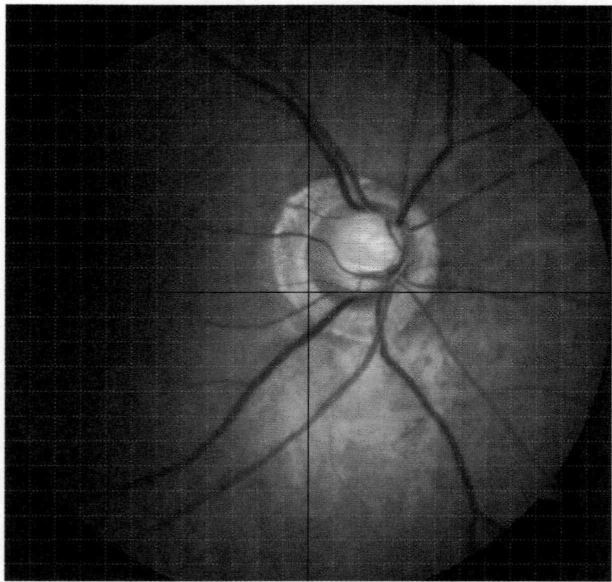

Average-large size nerve with diffuse parapapillary atrophy and diffuse neuroretinal rim thinning.

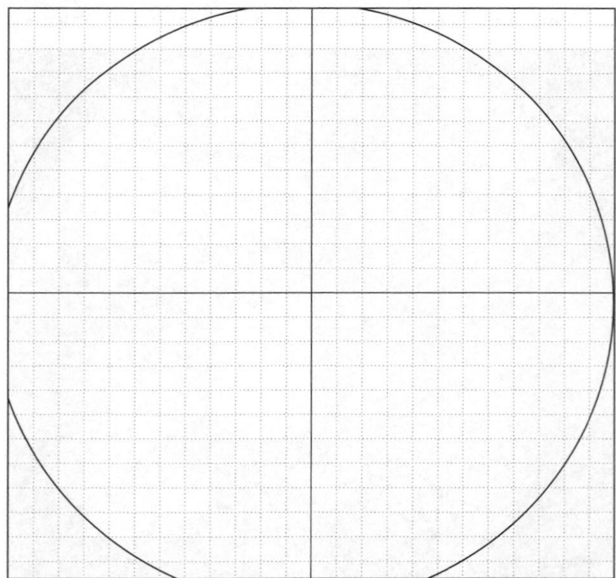

10. RETINAL ARTERIOLE DIAMETER

Overview

Progressive optic nerve damage (glaucomatous or nonglaucomatous) is associated with focal narrowing of the retinal arterioles and is proportional to the stage of the optic neuropathy.[1–3] Retinal arteriole narrowing is characteristic of, but not always specific for, glaucoma.[4]

Regarding glaucomatous optic nerve damage in all forms, the focal narrowing of the retinal arterioles is associated with decreased neuroretinal rim area, decreased retinal nerve fiber layer (RNFL) visibility, and increased associated visual field defects.[4] This vessel diameter narrowing may be due to autoregulation from decreased vascular demand in the superficial layers of the retina, and/or overall decreased optic nerve vascular perfusion (vascular insufficiency) common in patients with glaucoma.[4–6]

Pearls

- **Appearance:**
  - In the normal eyes, retinal arteriole diameters are widest at the temporal inferior disc, then temporal superior, then nasal superior area, and finally the nasal inferior disc region.[1,6]
    - Retinal arteriole diameters are independent of age, gender, or refractive error.[6]
    - Normal retinal arteriole diameter parallels or follows the same RNFL pattern distribution in normal eyes and the normal physiologic "ISNT rule" of the neuroretinal rim.
      - The diameter of the retinal arterioles in the normal eye may be proportional to the volume of tissue requiring perfusion.[6]
      - Vessel diameter decreases with corresponding decreasing area of the neuroretinal rim, diminishing visibility of the RNFL, and increasing visual field defects.
- **Significance:**
  - Typical of optic nerve damage but *not* necessarily pathognomonic for glaucoma.
    - Also found in other forms of nonglaucomatous optic neuropathies and in patients with advancing age.

- Severity of focal narrowing does not vary significantly between glaucomatous and nonglaucomatous optic nerve atrophy.
- Retinal arterials may be *more* narrow in eyes with normal-tension glaucoma and eyes with nonarteritic ischemic optic neuropathies than other groups.
  - As normal-tension glaucoma progresses, the retinal arteriole diameter decreases.[3,7]
- For glaucoma, the degree of focal narrowing of the retinal arterioles is significantly more pronounced if the optic nerve damage is more advanced.
- Glaucomatous visual field defects in primary open-angle glaucoma are associated with decreased diameter of the associated retinal arterioles in the corresponding hemifield.[8]
- Retinal arterial narrowing is a long-term risk factor for the development of primary open-angle glaucoma.[9]

References

1. Jonas JB, Budde WM, Panda-Jonas S. Ophthalmoscopic evaluation of the optic nerve head. *Surv Ophthalmol.* 1999;43:293–320.
2. Papastathopoulos K, Jonas J. Follow up of focal narrowing of retinal arterioles in glaucoma. *Br J Ophthalmol.* 1999;83(3):285–289.
3. Lee T, Kim Y, Yoo C. Retinal vessel diameter in normal-tension glaucoma patients with asymmetric progression. *Graefes Arch Clin Exp Ophthalmol.* 2014;252(11):1795–1801.
4. Papastathopoulos K, Jonas J. Fluorescein angiographic correlation of focal narrowing of retinal arterioles in glaucoma. *Br J Ophthalmol.* 1998;82(1):48–50.
5. Papastathopoulos K, Jonas J. Follow up of focal narrowing of retinal arterioles in glaucoma. *Br J Ophthalmol.* 1999;83(3):285–289.
6. Mitchell P, Leung H, Klein R, et al. Retinal vessel diameter and open-angle glaucoma. The Blue Mountains eye study. *Ophthalmology.* 2005;112:245–250.
7. Wang S, Xu L, Wang Y, et al. Retinal vessel diameter in normal and glaucomatous eyes: the Beijing eye study. *Clin Experiment Ophthalmol.* 2007;35(9):800–807.
8. Hall J, Andrews A, Walker R, et al. Association of retinal vessel caliber and visual field defects in glaucoma. *Am J Ophthalmol.* 2001;132:855–859.
9. Kawasaki R, Wang J, Rochtchina E, et al. Retinal vessel caliber is associated with the 10-year incidence of glaucoma. The Blue Mountains eye study. *Ophthalmology.* 2013;120:84–90.

Further Reading

1. Kurvinen L, Kytö J, Summanen P, et al. Change in retinal blood flow and retinal arterial diameter after intraocular pressure reduction in glaucomatous eyes. *Acta Ophthalmol.* 2014;92(6):507.

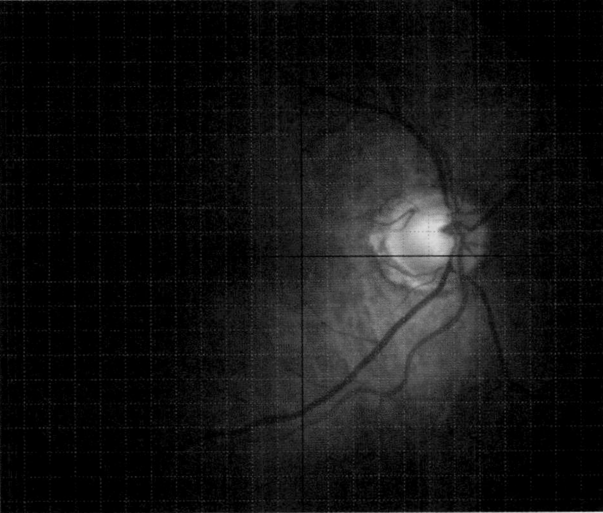

Average size nerve with neuroretinal rim thinning and associated retinal arteriole narrowing.

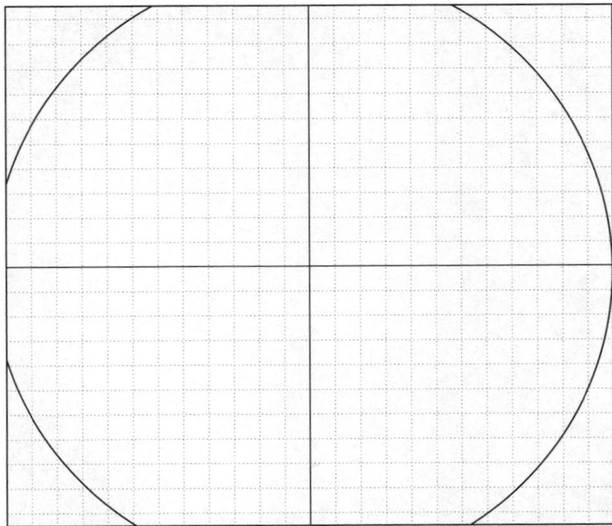

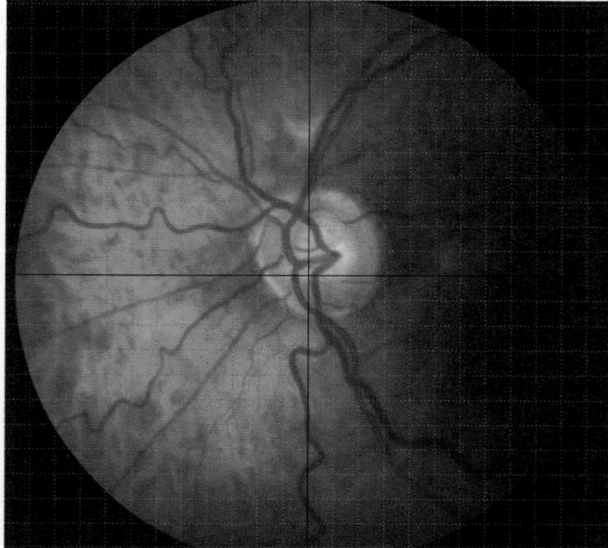

Average size nerve with vertical neuroretinal rim thinning and associated retinal arteriole narrowing.

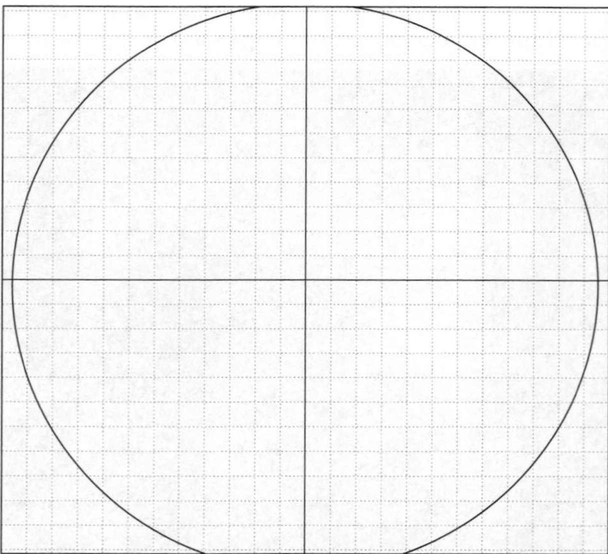

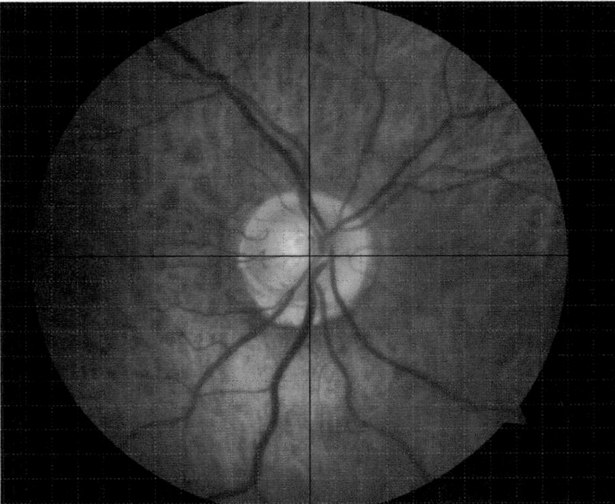

Average size nerve with inferior neuroretinal rim thinning, inferior parapapillary atrophy, and associated retinal arteriole narrowing.

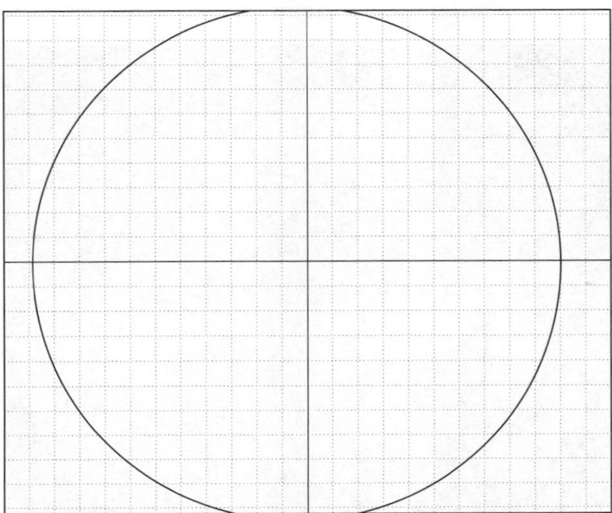

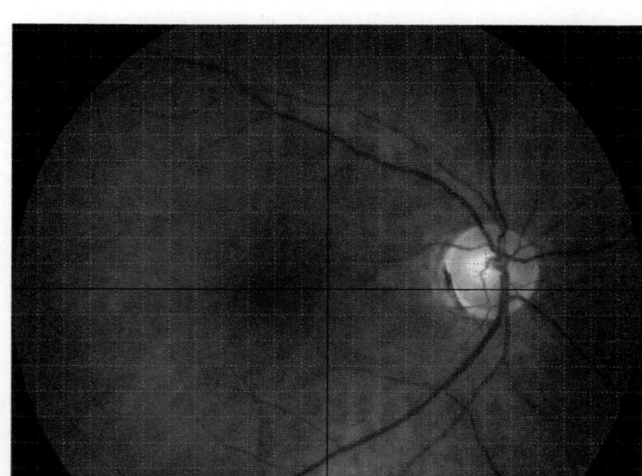

Average size nerve with inferior neuroretinal rim thinning, inferior parapapillary atrophy, and associated retinal arteriole narrowing.

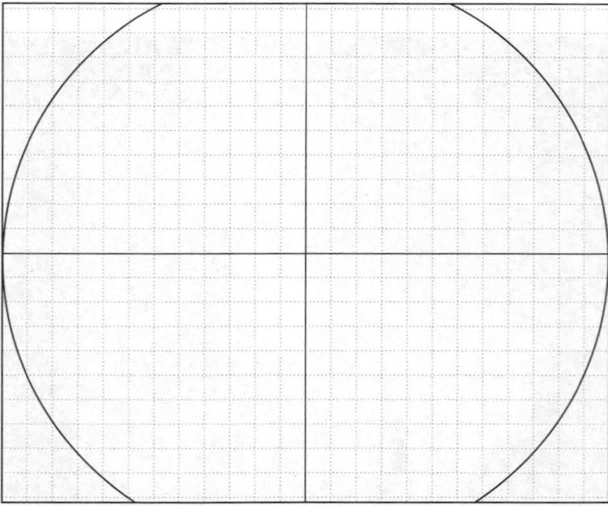

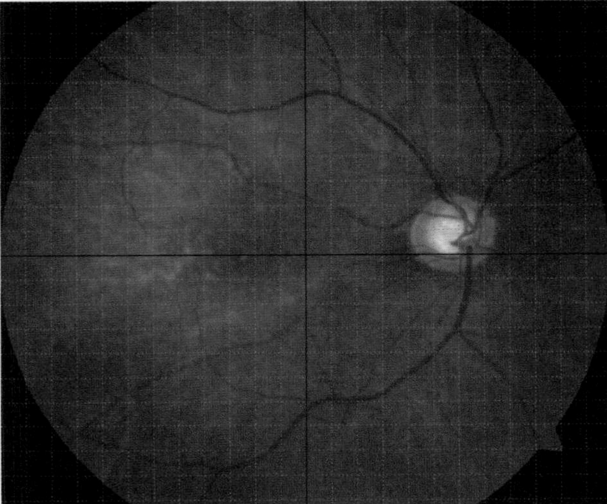

Average size nerve with superior neuroretinal rim thinning and associated retinal arteriole narrowing.

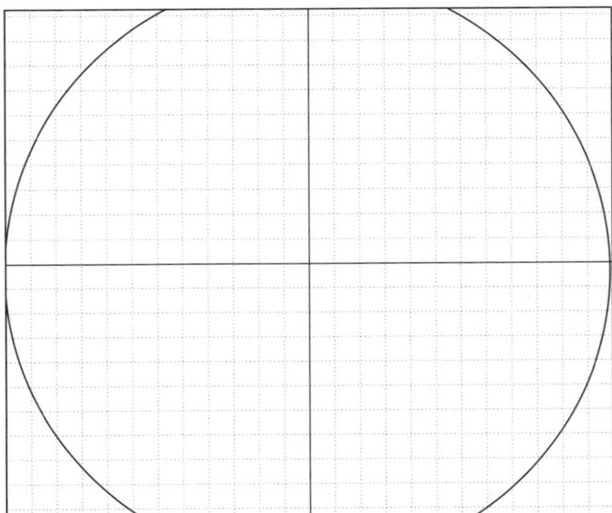

11. RETINAL NERVE FIBER LAYER DEFECTS

Overview

The retinal nerve fiber layer (RNFL) is composed of retinal ganglion cell axons that are covered by astrocytes and bundled by Muller cell processes.[1]

Glaucoma is a progressive optic neuropathy with characteristic and relative accelerated RNFL loss with associated morphologic changes to the optic nerve.[2,3] Localized RNFL defects are some of the earliest signs of glaucoma (average of 39% to 59% fewer retinal ganglion cells than age-matched normal subject)[3–5] and are less likely to be observed in advanced glaucoma due to diffuse RNFL loss and progression.[1,3] Such localized RNFL defects represent substantial amounts of retinal ganglion cell loss in the affected sector (even in the presence of normal visual fields) and are most common in the inferotemporal region followed by the superotemporal region.[3–5]

Careful evaluation of the optic nerve complex in the inferotemporal and superotemporal regions for RNFL defects may be more sensitive than visual field testing in those already diagnosed with early glaucoma.[6] The rate of RNFL loss appears to be faster (more than twice as fast) in glaucoma suspect patients who developed visual field defects than those who did not develop visual field defects.[7]

Pearls

- **Appearance:**
  - The visibility of the normal RNFL pattern and any potential localized RNFL defects depend on the race, age, and stage of the disease of the patient.[1,3]
    - Visibility of the RNFL decreases with age.
      - 1.4 million optic nerve fibers to start, loses about 4,000 to 5,000 fibers per year with normal aging process.
    - Appears as bright, fine striations in the inner retinal layer fanning off of the optic disc to the retinal periphery.
      - Easier to visualize with red-free filter and clear media.
      - Minor defects may be better seen on photographs.
  - Clinical findings in normal eyes:
    - Uneven distribution pattern over eight regions:
      - (Most visible) temporal/inferior > temporal/superior > nasal/superior > nasal/inferior > superior > inferior > temporal/horizontal > nasal/horizontal (least visible).

- Clinical findings in glaucomatous eyes:
  - Localized RNFL loss:
    - Wedge defects: narrow or broad localized defects that radiate outward *from* the optic disc border.
      - Often found 6 to 8 weeks after optic disc hemorrhages.
      - *Points* to localized neuroretinal rim loss and is adjacent to the optic disc border.
        - Pseudo-localized wedge defects:
          - Do not completely extend to the optic disc border.
          - Do not have a broad base close to the temporal horizontal raphe of the fundus.
      - Visible localized defects represent substantial RNFL loss.
    - Noted in about 20% of all glaucoma eyes.
      - Frequency increases significantly from early glaucoma to moderate glaucoma and *then* decreases with advanced glaucoma.
      - More common in focal-type normal-tension glaucoma than in eyes with age-related atrophic open-angle glaucoma (OAG), highly myopic OAG, and juvenile-onset OAG.
      - Most often found in the temporal inferior sector followed by the temporal superior sector
        - Rarely noted in nasal fundus region.
      - *Not* pathognomonic for glaucoma.
        - Observed in optic nerve atrophy due to optic disc drusen, toxoplasmosis scars, ischemic retinopathies, post chronic papilledema, and optic neuritis.
          - Likely nonglaucomatous optic atrophy if:
            - Decreased RNFL visibility.
            - Decreased retinal arteriole diameter.
            - Increased optic nerve pallor.
            - Stable parapapillary atrophy.
        - Low sensitivity because of relatively low frequency in eyes with optic nerve damage.
        - Localized RNFL defects NOT present in normal eyes.
          - Important application in patients with ocular hypertension who may have normal perimetric testing.
  - Diffuse RNFL loss:
    - More difficult to detect than localized loss but look for:
      - *Less* visible RNFL in the temporal inferior fundus region *compared to* the temporal superior fundus region (assuming no fundus irregularities).
        - Intraocular and interocular comparison necessary to detect subtle relative RNFL pattern loss.

- Increased retinal vessel clarity.
  - ◇ Important variable in the diagnosis of optic nerve damage.

- **Significance:**
  - The RNFL should be carefully and systematically examined during every routine exam.
  - One of the *earliest* signs of glaucomatous optic nerve damage and is especially helpful for:
    - Pseudo-normal but glaucomatous average cups in smaller nerves.
    - Pseudo-glaucomatous *but* normal large cup in larger nerves.
      - ○ Less helpful in advanced disease.

References

1. Jonas JB, Budde WM, Panda-Jonas S. Ophthalmoscopic evaluation of the optic nerve head. *Surv Ophthalmol.* 1999;43:293–320.
2. Weinreb R, Aung T, Medeiros F. The pathophysiology and treatment of glaucoma: a review. *JAMA.* 2014;311(18):1901–1911.
3. Tatham A, Weinreb R, Zangwill L, et al. Estimated retinal ganglion cell counts in glaucomatous eyes with localized retinal nerve fiber layer defects. *Am J Ophthalmol.* 2013;156(3):578–587.e1.
4. Quigley HA. Examination of the retinal nerve fiber layer in the recognition of early glaucoma damage. *Trans Am Ophthalmol Soc.* 1986;84:920–966.
5. Sommer A, Katz J, Quigley HA, et al. Clinically detectable nerve fiber atrophy precedes the onset of glaucomatous field loss. *Arch Ophthalmol.* 1991;109(1):77–83.
6. Alasil T, Wang K, Chen T, et al. Correlation of retinal nerve fiber layer thickness and visual fields in glaucoma: a broken stick model. *Am J Ophthalmol.* 2014;157:953–959.e2.
7. Miki A, Medeiros F, Zangwill L, et al. Rates of retinal nerve fiber layer thinning in glaucoma suspect eyes. *Ophthalmology.* 2014;121:1350–1358.

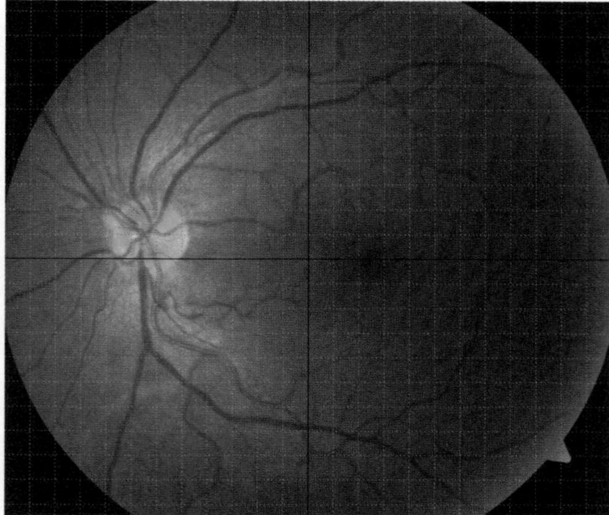

Average-small size nerve with bright, robust retinal nerve fiber layer (RNFL) pattern. Note: Normal diminished vessel clarity inferiorly and superiorly due to healthy and preserved RNFL density. In general, retinal vessel clarity is indirectly proportional to RNFL density.

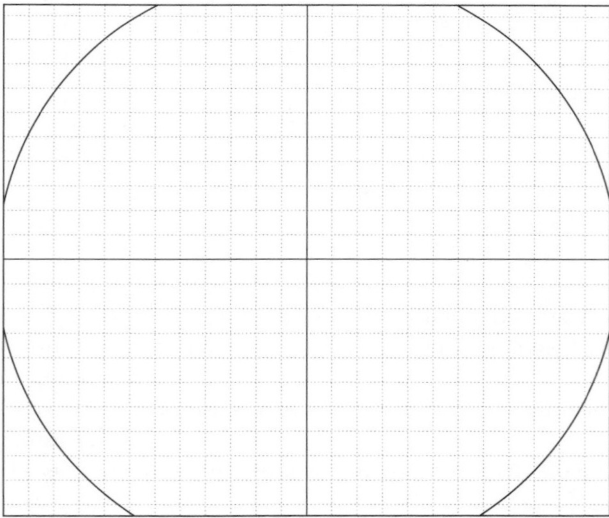

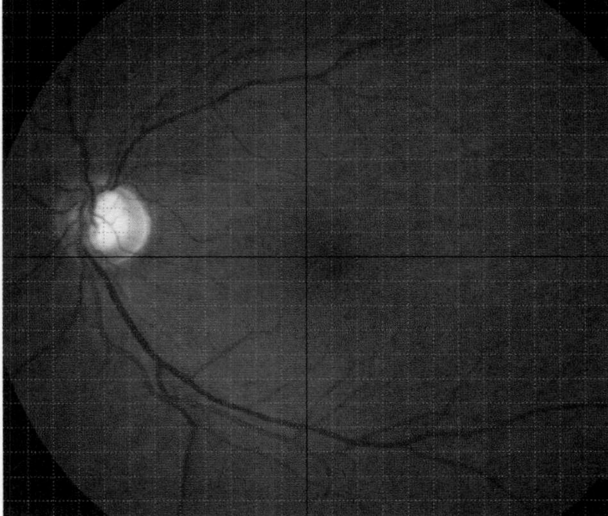

Average size nerve with superior temporal thinning and associated diffuse retinal nerve fiber layer loss. Note: Increased superior vessel clarity relative to inferior vessels.

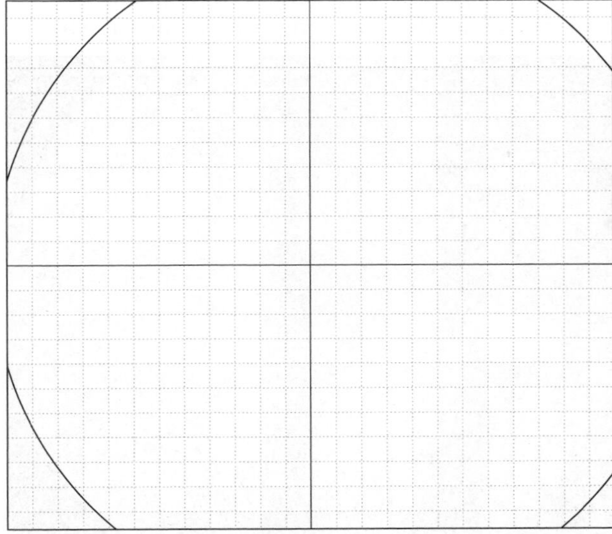

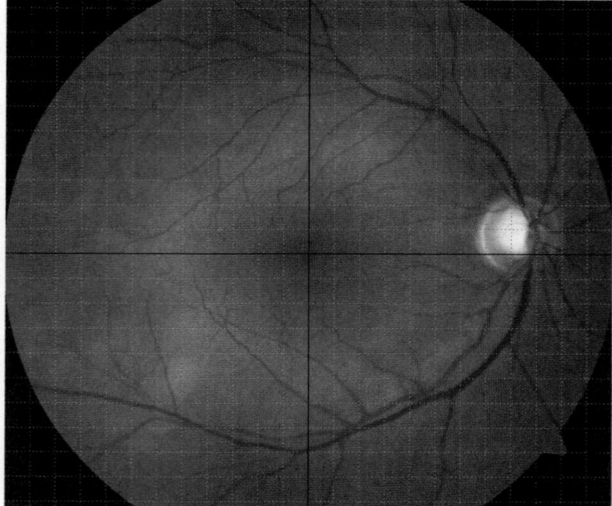

Average size nerve with superior temporal thinning and associated diffuse retinal nerve fiber layer loss. Note: Increased superior vessel clarity relative to inferior vessels.

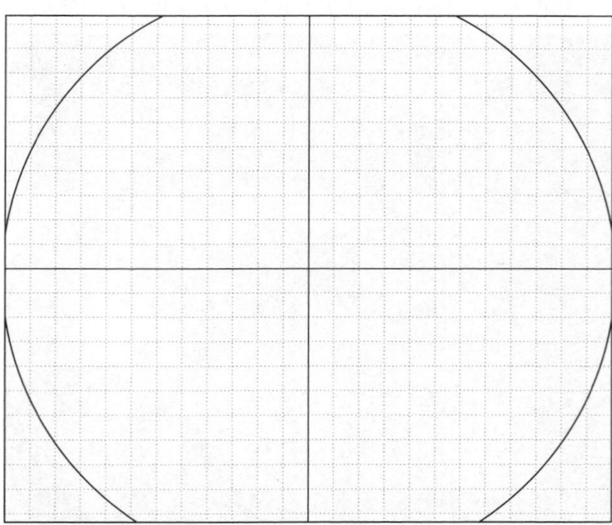

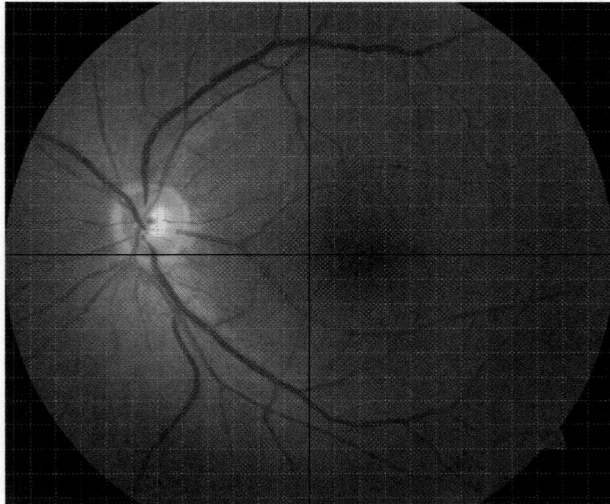

Average-small size nerve with superior-temporal neuroretinal rim thinning and associated localized retinal nerve fiber layer defects.

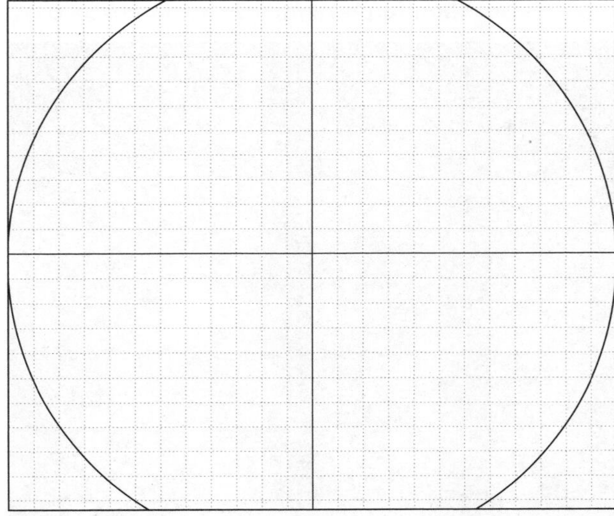

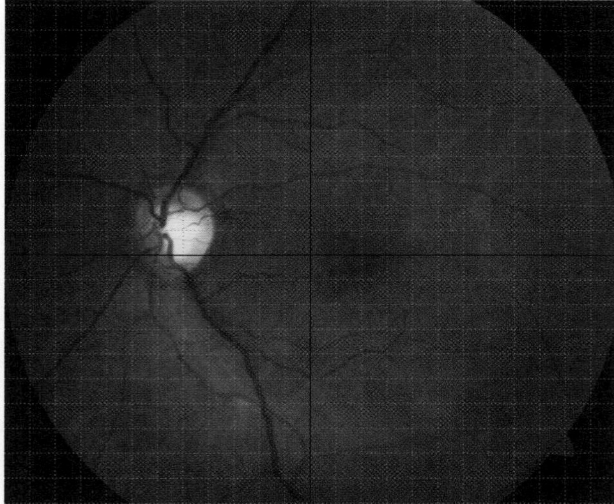

Average size nerve with inferior thinning, associated localized retinal nerve fiber layer loss, and increased inferior vessel clarity.

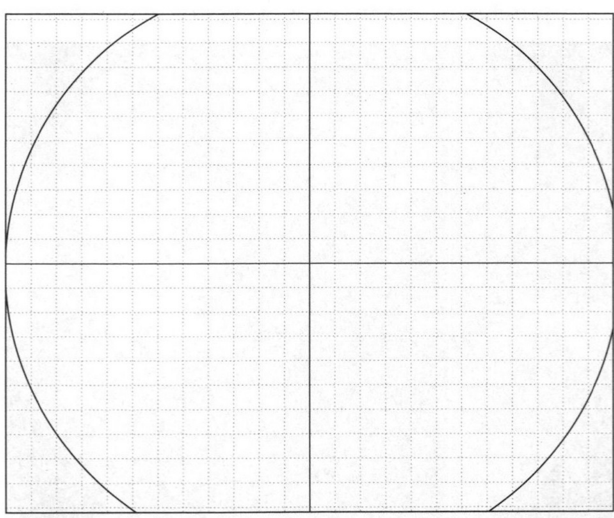

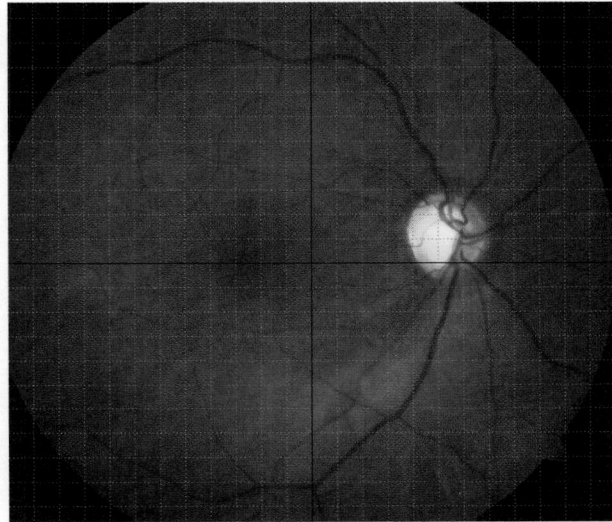

Average size nerve with inferior thinning and associated localized retinal nerve fiber layer loss.

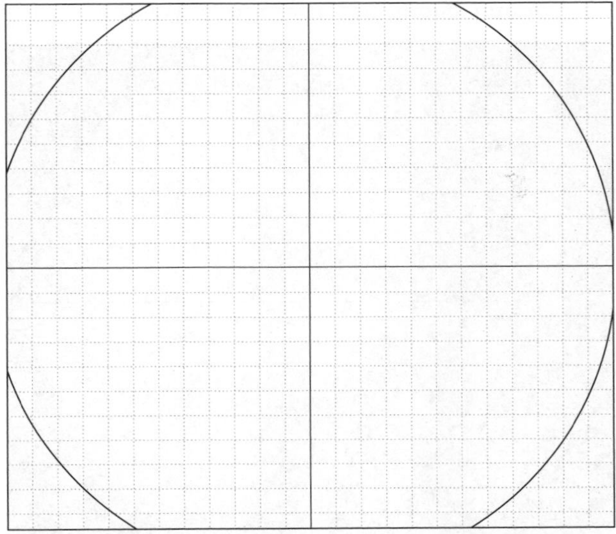

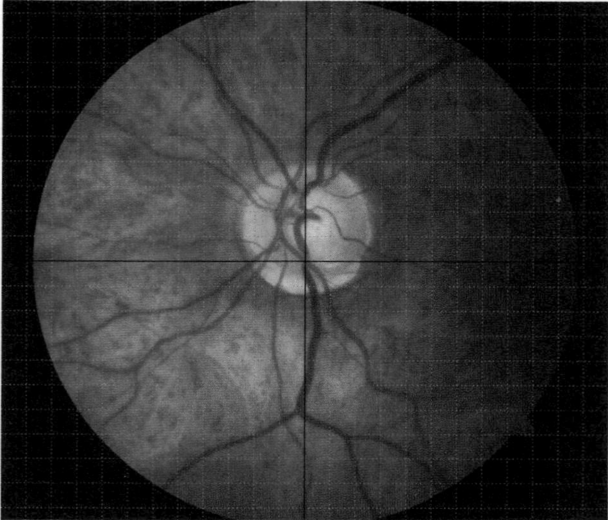

Average size nerve with vertical thinning, inferior parapapillary atrophy, diffuse retinal nerve fiber layer loss, and relative increased vessel clarity.

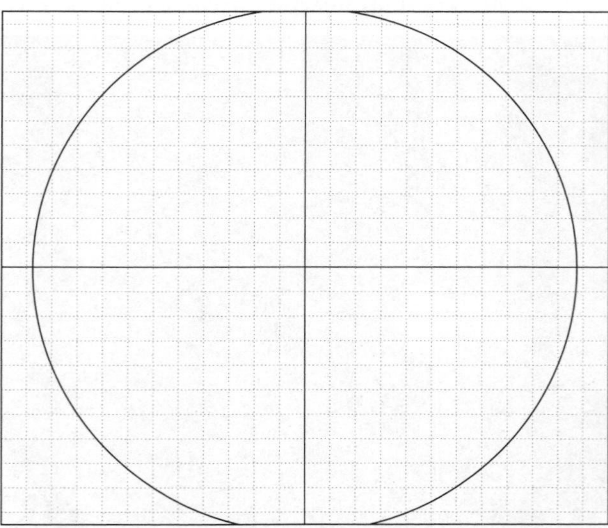

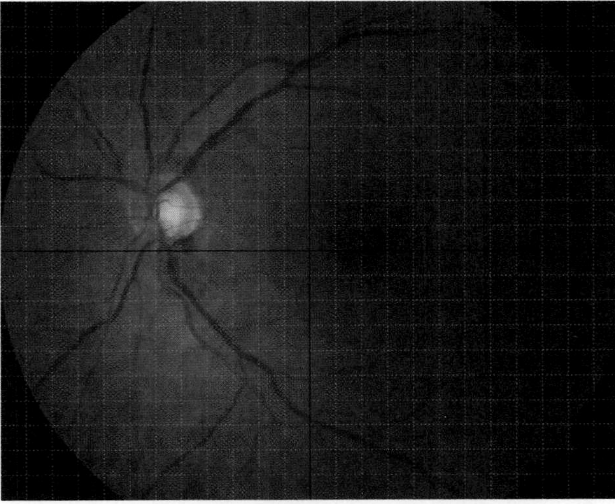

Average-small nerve with inferior neuroretinal rim thinning, inferior localized retinal nerve fiber layer defect, and associated adjacent glaucomatous disc hemorrhage.

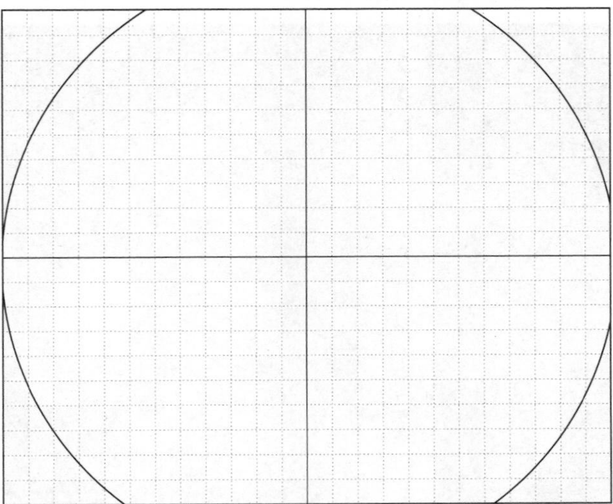

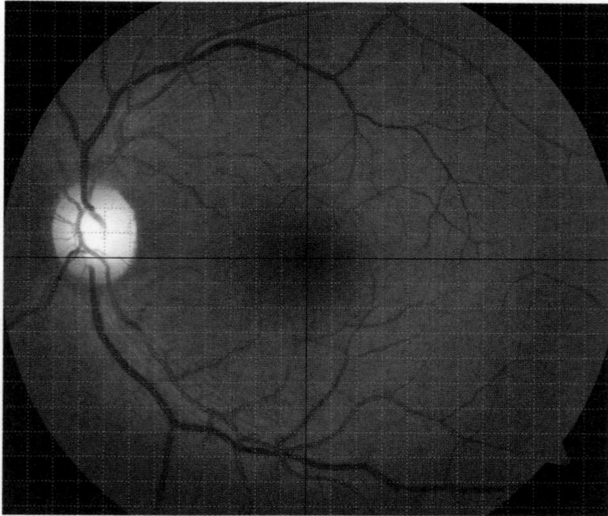

Average-large size nerve with healthy retinal nerve fiber layer appearance.

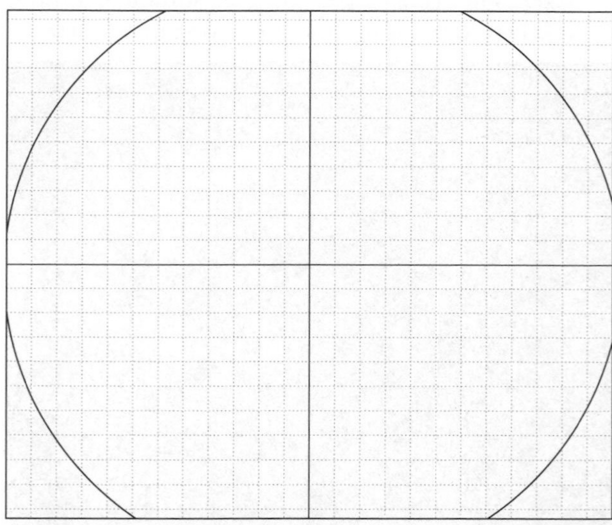

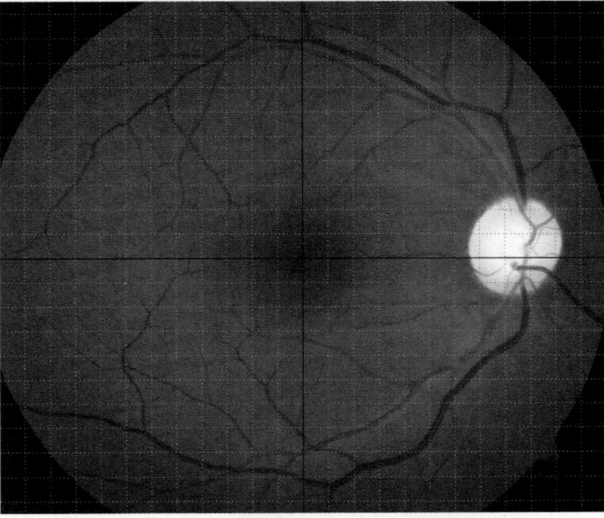

Average size nerve with superior temporal localized retinal nerve fiber layer defects.

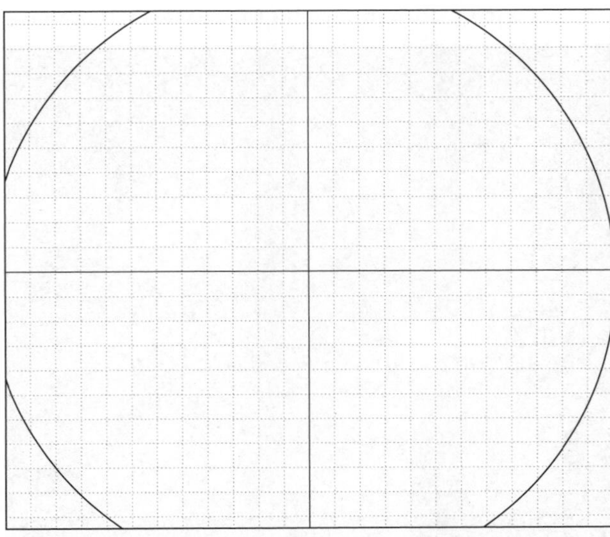

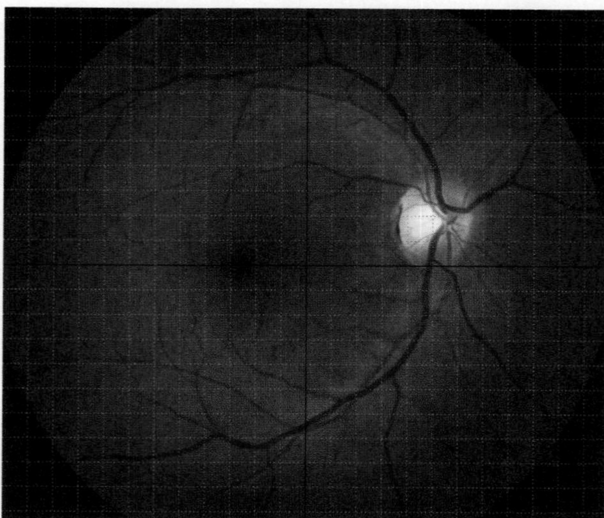

Average size nerve with inferior neuroretinal rim thinning, inferior diffuse retinal nerve fiber layer loss, and relative increased inferior vessel clarity.

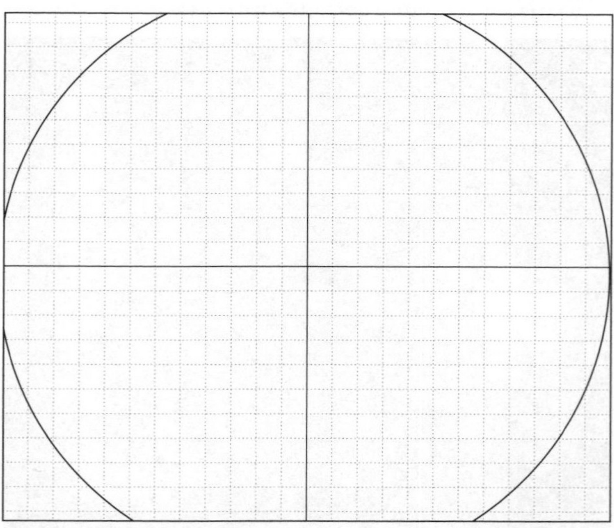

12. CONCLUSION

Several factors can help to differentiate between glaucomatous and nonglaucomatous optic neuropathy.[1–3]

- **Glaucomatous optic neuropathy is associated with:**
  - Older age.
  - Elevated intraocular pressures.
  - Thinner pachymetry.
  - Visual acuity better than 20/40.
  - Minimal if any neuroretinal rim pallor.
    - Pallor has been reported in glaucomatous optic neuropathy.
    - Pallor may initially be absent in nonglaucomatous optic neuropathy.
  - Greater cup-disc ratio with vertical elongation.
    - Focal or diffuse neuroretinal rim loss (87% specific).
  - Greater frequency of parapapillary atrophy.
    - Nonglaucomatous optic neuropathy usually does NOT have parapapillary atrophy and, if it does, it does not usually progress.
  - Optic disc hemorrhage.
    - The *presence* of optic disc hemorrhages is more significant or meaningful than the *absence* of optic disc hemorrhages.
  - Family history of glaucoma.
  - Visual field defects that respect more the horizontal meridian.

- **Nonglaucomatous optic neuropathy is associated with:**
  - Younger age (<50 years of age).
  - Visual acuity worse than 20/40.
  - Pallor that exceeds or extends beyond the cupping (94% specific).
  - Visual field defects that respect more the vertical meridian.

Glaucomatous and nonglaucomatous optic neuropathy may *share* the following morphologic features:

- **Decreased retinal arteriole diameter with focal arteriole narrowing.**
- **Reduced retinal nerve fiber layer (RNFL) visibility.**
- **Localized RNFL defects.**
- **Enlargement and deepening of optic cup.**
  - Correlating decreased neuroretinal rim thickness.

The most important variables for diagnosing early glaucoma include the following[1]:

- **Shape and width of neuroretinal rim:**
  - The rim shape is influenced by the location of the central retinal vessel trunk.
  - Inferior and superior rim width should be relatively broader when compared with the temporal disc region.
    - Consider glaucoma suspect IF the neuroretinal rim is of equal width in all disc regions.
- **Size of the optic cup in relation to the size of the optic disc.**
  - An average size cup in a smaller nerve may be more suspicious for glaucoma than a larger size cup in a larger nerve.
- **Localized or diffuse-decreased RNFL visibility and correlating increased vessel clarity.**
- **Presence of optic disc hemorrhages.**

References

1. Jonas JB, Budde WM, Panda-Jonas S. Ophthalmoscopic evaluation of the optic nerve head. *Surv Ophthalmol.* 1999;43:293–320.
2. Choudhari N, Neog A, Fudnawala V, et al. Cupped disc with normal intraocular pressure: the long road to avoid misdiagnosis. *Indian J Ophthalmol.* 2011;59(6):491–497.
3. Greenfield D, Siatkowski R, Glaser J, et al. The cupped disc. Who needs neuroimaging? *Ophthalmology.* 1998;105(10):1866–1874.

Index